Finding Happiness Through Pain And Embarrassment

My Life With Behcet's Disease – A Memoir

Also By Ellis Michaels

Inside Out (Bloodfeast Book 1)

Back In The Game (Bloodfeast Book 2)

The Final Quest (Bloodfeast Book 3)

Ordinary Hero

Bad Unicorn

Ellis Michaels Website

ellismichaels.com

Finding Happiness Through Pain And Embarrassment

My Life With Behcet's Disease –
A Memoir

by **Ellis Michaels**

Infinite Summer Publishing, LLC

SOME NAMES HAVE BEEN CHANGED TO PROTECT THE
PRIVACY OF INDIVIDUALS. OTHERS HAVE BEEN
CHANGED TO PROTECT THE AUTHOR FROM GETTING
SUED FOR CALLING PEOPLE NOT-SO-NICE NAMES.

COPYRIGHT 2020 © ELLIS MICHAELS

FIRST INFINITE SUMMER PUBLISHING EDITION
DECEMBER 2020

ISBN: 978-1-7333240-3-8

Dedicated to anyone who's recently been diagnosed with Behcet's disease – or any chronic illness, for that matter.

You may, at times, suffer in solitude. But you'll never suffer alone.

Table of Contents

Introduction.............................. 1
1. Diagnosed............................ 9
2. Little Red Bumps..................... 18
3. Acne................................. 26
4. Sores................................ 32
5. Knee Surgery......................... 40
6. Retinitis............................ 49
7. Denial............................... 56
8. Sacked............................... 63
9. Clot................................. 70
10. Rock & Roll......................... 81
11. Drained............................. 88
12. Loneliness.......................... 96
13. Brown............................... 101
14. Sex & Drugs......................... 107
15. Broken.............................. 115
16. Fixed............................... 126
17. Damaged............................. 134
18. Negative To Positive................ 141
19. No Sex & No Drugs................... 148
20. The Dark Ages....................... 155
21. Labyrinth........................... 163
22. Not Again........................... 169
23. Doctor, Doctor...................... 176
24. Write............................... 184
25. Stomach Pain on the Fourth.......... 191
26. The Summer of Acceptance............ 197
27. Back In Action...................... 203
28. Clot Again.......................... 209
29. Breaking Up......................... 217
30. Olivia.............................. 227
31. 2020 Vision......................... 236
32. Attitude............................ 244

From The Author
Acknowledgments
More From Ellis Michaels

Introduction

Mystery pain. That's what I used to call it when I was a kid. I never knew why it happened or when it would happen next. The only thing I knew for sure was that, sooner or later, it would be happening again.

Sometimes it'd be my stomach. Out of nowhere it would feel like I swallowed a swarm of angry wasps. One minute I'd be fine. The next minute I'd be curled up in a ball on my bedroom floor in tears.

Sometimes it would be my joints. For no apparent reason they'd swell up like a balloon. It might be one of my knees or elbows. It might be a few of my fingers. Whatever joints were swollen, they hurt.

Sometimes it would be my mouth. Before I'd even hit puberty, I started getting big, quarter-sized ulcers in my mouth and on my tongue. Those were the worst. They'd be so painful that it hurt to eat, brush my teeth, and even talk.

If it wasn't one strange, painful symptom, it'd be another. Mystery pain was a regular part of my childhood. The pain itself was awful. But that wasn't the worst part. The worst was the mystery of it all. As a kid, I had no idea why my body was causing itself so much pain and neither did my parents or my pediatrician.

But I do now.

I was diagnosed with Behcet's disease at the age of sixteen. After a decade of unexplained symptoms, I finally learned the name of what had been causing them. I was relieved to have a diagnosis – an explanation for my suffering. But the more I learned about it, the more terrified I became.

Behcet's is an autoimmune disease – one of many. Even if you've never heard of it, you probably *have* heard of some other autoimmune diseases. There are over a hundred of them altogether. Lupus, Crohn's, Fibromyalgia, MS, and rheumatoid arthritis are some of the more well-known varieties. But there are plenty of others.

Autoimmune diseases affect roughly 15-million Americans or about 5% of the population.[1] That means the odds of having *some* autoimmune condition is about one in twenty. Behcet's disease affects roughly 3,600 Americans or 0.001% of the population.[2] The odds of having Behcet's is roughly one in three-hundred thousand. That means you're about ten times more likely to get struck by lightening than to have Behcet's disease. Lucky me.

With all autoimmune diseases, the body attacks itself. Instead of just fighting off foreign invaders like it's supposed to, the immune system also attacks perfectly health tissue. *What* tissue depends on the specific illness. Some autoimmune diseases only affect one part of the body while others can wreak havoc on multiple systems. Crohn's, for example, only hits the gastrointestinal tract from your mouth to your butt. Something like Lupus, however, can affect everything from your skin to your lungs, your brain to your bones.

Behcet's really only causes inflammation in

---

[1] Hayter, S., & Cook, M. (2012). Updated assessment of the prevalence, spectrum and case definition of autoimmune disease. *Autoimmunity Reviews*, 11(10):754-65.

[2] Estimates of prevalence for autoimmune disease. (n.d.). *Autoimmune Registry, Inc.* Retrieved September 21, 2020 from https://www.autoimmuneregistry.org/autoimmune-statistics

one body part: blood vessels. But guess where blood vessels are? Everywhere. They're in your heart, lungs, eyes, ears, muscles, skin, brain, and anywhere else there's living tissue. So Behcet's can affect just about any part of the body, head to toe. Some common symptoms include painful oral and genital ulcers, arthritis, eye problems, and fatigue. Less common but more serious, Behcet's can cause blood clots, aneurysms, blindness, deafness, paralysis, and even death. And that's only a sample of potential symptoms. There are plenty more.

If you sat down and tried to come up with the most-painful-and-embarrassing-yet-largely-invisible illness you possibly could, it would probably look a lot like Behcet's disease. There's really only one way to describe living with it:

Having Behcet's disease fucking sucks.

If I could snap my fingers and make this illness magically disappear, I'd do it in a heartbeat. I wouldn't wish it upon my worst enemy. Living with Behcet's disease is a relentless struggle, a constant battle against your own body. You never know when or where the next attack is coming. Any given day could be the day I lose my vision forever. Today could be the day I lose my hearing or my ability to walk. It might even be the day I take my last breath. So I stand by my former statement: Behcet's sucks.

But it's not all bad.

Okay, I'm not going to lie: it's *mostly* bad. But believe it or not, there are silver linings to having a painful, unpredictable, havoc-wreaking, lifelong illness. Positive things can come out of negative experiences. Sometimes you have to look really, *really* hard to find that positivity. But it's always there if you look hard enough for it.

And that's exactly what I've done. No matter how lousy I've felt physically, how exhausted and depressed I've felt mentally, how broke I've felt financially, or how lonely I've felt socially, I've learned to focus on the positive. And if I've looked hard enough – sometimes really, *really* hard – I've always found it.

My life would be a lot different if I didn't have Behcet's disease. I wouldn't have scars all over my body, varicose veins popping out of my legs and abs, and I'd likely still have a mouth full of my own natural teeth. My days wouldn't have to begin and end with me downing a handful of pills from the small pharmacy I keep on my nightstand. I wouldn't have to see four specialists and get eight vials of blood drawn every six months. My past wouldn't be nearly as riddled with pain, suffering, and embarrassment as it has been. And I'd no longer have to worry about my future plans being sabotaged by my own treasonous body.

But if I didn't have Behcet's, my life would also be different in a number of less-positive ways. For one, I wouldn't know what Behcet's disease is. I probably wouldn't even know what autoimmune diseases are in general. I wouldn't know any of the fascinating things I've learned from studying my malfunctioning body for over two decades. I've learned a ton about health, fitness, nutrition, medicine, and psychology that I wouldn't have if I'd never been diagnosed with Behcet's. But the knowledge I've acquired from having this lousy illness is only one of its silver linings.

If I didn't have Behcet's disease, I never would've swam with dolphins. I wouldn't have kayaked down the countless miles of rivers, mountain climbed the countless feet of elevation, or traveled the countless miles around the world that I have. I wouldn't have quit a job I hated to start building my dream career. And I wouldn't have the courage to get up and pursue my dreams with all I've got every single day.

Believe it or not, Behcet's disease has given me all these things. It's motivated me to get as much out of life as I possibly can *while* I still can. Knowing I could lose my vision, hearing, mobility, or even my life at any moment has lit a brightly burning fire under my ass that keeps me moving forward at all times. There are so many fun and interesting things to do in this world and we only get so much time to do them. That's true for *all* of us. The clock is always ticking. But when you're living with a disease like Behcet's, that clock is ticking in double time.

My illness has forced me to learn things I'd never know otherwise. It's pushed me to travel the world and live life to the fullest. But I still haven't mentioned the greatest silver lining of having Behcet's disease.

It's *you*.

It's the wonderful friends I've made along the way. It's the other Behcet's sufferers I've developed deep, meaningful relationships with. It's the awesome online communities of people living with Behcet's and other chronic illnesses who regularly go out of their way to help each other. It's the connections I've made with people from all over the world who I never would've met if I didn't have this shitty illness. And yes, it's you – *you personally* – the one holding this book. The person I get the privilege of sharing my story with. If I didn't have Behcet's disease, I wouldn't have written this book and you wouldn't be reading it.

That's the theme I'm going for in this memoir: the silver linings of living with Behcet's or any other chronic disease. It's fitting, since one of the main themes of my adult life has been turning negatives into positives. But I'm not going to sugarcoat anything. Having Behcet's disease totally sucks and I'll make no attempt to hide that fact. I'll be going into detail about the horrors of living with a body that's constantly trying to harm itself. I'm going to tell you about the massive ulcers I used to get in my mouth and on my balls; the severe inflammation I had in one of my eyes that almost left me permanently blind; the embarrassment of going through high school with golf-ball-sized cysts all over my face; the pain of having clots in both legs and other parts of my body; the loneliness, anxiety, and depression that go along with having a rare illness; the failure of the American medical system to help people like me; the addiction to painkillers I developed in my teens; and even the time I was so fed up with it all that I actually tried to kill myself. And that's just the tip of the iceberg.

But it's also only half of the story.

I've learned to take the pain, suffering, loneliness, depression, anxiety, embarrassment, and everything else this illness has thrown at me and turn it all around. I've learned to find the silver lining in every symptom and every setback. I've taken all the negatives of living with Behcet's disease and turned them into positives. In this memoir, I'm going to show you how I did it and how you can, too.

In spite of my diagnosis, in spite of all the pain and suffering, I've lived an awesome life. I've learned to see the good in the bad, the positive in the negative, the light in the darkness. But the operative word is *learned*. Positivity does not come naturally to me and it never has. It takes effort. Sometimes *a lot* of effort. But in the end, it's been so fucking worth it.

This is a story about what it's like to live with Behcet's disease. It's also a story of personal transformation. A story of hope for anyone who's recently been diagnosed with Behcet's or any other chronic illness. A story of encouragement for anyone who wants to be more positive, regardless of whether they have a chronic illness or not. A story of what's possible with the right attitude and a willingness to change.

This is *my* story. It hasn't been easy putting it out there for the world to see and judge. Those who know me best know I'm a mostly private person. Openly talking about sores on my balls or trying to off myself are not things I'm very comfortable blabbing about in public. In a private conversation, sure. Not in a book for all the world to see. But I forced myself to leap outside of my comfort zone and write this book in the hope that some*one* some*where* will benefit from it some*how*. I knew that could only happen by being totally honest and leaving nothing out no matter how embarrassing. So that's exactly what I've written: an honest memoir about the good, the bad, and the downright embarrassing of living with Behcet's disease.

Lastly, I've done my best to write this story in my own voice, the same way you'd hear me tell it in real life. Originally, I considered writing this as a light-and-fluffy PG-rated memoir. But Behcet's isn't a light-and-fluffy illness – and it certainly ain't PG. So I'm not going to censor myself. I'm going to write the way I talk, using the same language and everything. And sometimes when I speak, especially when discussing all the suffering Behcet's disease has caused me, a swear[1] or two are bound to come out every once in a while. I try not to overdo the profanity, but beware there is some language in this memoir that might not be suitable for sensitive readers. And there is subject matter some people may find distasteful. But again, Behcet's is a distasteful disease. It can't be discussed – not in an open and honest way – without talking about some pretty disturbing things. So if you're offended by topics like sex, drugs, suicide, or genital ulcers, this memoir isn't for you. Same with swears. If an occasional f-bomb bothers you, this book ain't for you. The last thing I want to do is offend anyone unnecessarily. So if this memoir ain't your cup o' tea, go find something else to read. I won't hold it against you.

But I hope you decide to stick around. If you do, it means the world to me that you're giving this book a chance. To most, it's just another memoir, one among thousands published every year. But to me this *was*, *is*, and *always will be* my life. Here's the story of how I managed to find happiness through the pain and embarrassment of living with Behcet's disease. Enjoy.

Ellis Michaels
October 24, 2020

---

[1] Or for my wonderful Southern and Midwestern readers, a cuss word or two are bound to come out.

"The truth," Dumbledore sighed. "It's a beautiful and terrible thing, and should therefore be treated with great caution." - J.K. Rowling (from Harry Potter and the Sorcerer's Stone)

1. Diagnosed

Attitude is everything. It can be the difference between success and failure. Between happiness and misery. A positive attitude will open doors and keep you moving forward even when things are at their worst. It will do more for you than just about anything else in the world. A negative one will hold you back, keep you miserable, and make you feel like a constant failure.

My attitude used to be negative as hell.

By the time I hit my early teens, I'd already developed a round-the-clock bad attitude. I didn't get along with either of my parents, I hated school most of the time, and I kept having these weird symptoms all over my body. Some of them were wicked painful. Others were just embarrassing. But the worst part was not knowing the cause. Something wasn't right: that much was obvious. But I didn't know what and neither did my parents who were both experienced nurses. Even my pediatrician had no idea what was wrong with me.

It's one thing to have something bad happen to you. Having bad things happen to you regularly is something else. Having bad things happen to you regularly *for no apparent reason* is something different entirely. You've got nowhere to point your finger. Nothing to blame. No one to hold accountable. It leaves you feeling vulnerable and afraid, always wondering what the next unexplained symptom will be and when it'll happen.

Will it be painful? How painful? Will it be something others can see? Will I be embarrassed by it? Will it prevent me from doing things I like to do? Will it be temporary or will it cause permanent damage? Is there anything I can do to prevent it? Is there something I'm currently doing that will cause it? Is this my fault? Is this happening to me because I'm a bad person? Did I do something to deserve this?

My teens were filled with anxiety. I used to ask these questions and a thousand more all the time. The constant dread gradually eroded my spirit until I could only see darkness. Pessimism and negativity dominated my thoughts. There was no light at the end of the tunnel, no end to my suffering in sight. I had no confidence and even less self-esteem. What I *did* have was attitude and lots of it. But it wasn't the good kind that opens doors and breeds success. My attitude was terrible and I made no attempt at hiding it.

My poor parents caught the brunt of my negativity. For years I gave 'em hell. My anxiety often came out as anger and it was usually directed at them. My parents were even more anxious than me. Something was causing their firstborn son's body to attack itself and they had no idea what. My parents felt as powerless as I did and it ate away at all of us for years. But at the age of sixteen, all that changed when I met an ophthalmologist in Boston named Dr. Scott Woods.

* * *

All professions have their assholes. But other than maybe politics, I can't think of a profession more arrogance packed than medicine. Even the most humble of doctors can get a little cocky now and then. It comes with the territory. When you're trained to make life-or-death decisions, how could it not?

The most arrogant doctor I've ever met also happens to be the one I'm most thankful for. To this day he remains the most pompous, pretentious, and overall unpleasant MD I've ever dealt with. In some weird way that's actually a compliment. Over the years I've been to dozens of doctors in about ten different specialties. Some of them have been jerks, for sure. Many were stuck up, rude, and impatient. But none of them talked down to me with the same level of self-importance and condescension that *he* did.

"Sit still," Dr. Woods said, making no attempt to hide his frustration.

"It really hurts," I replied, making no attempt to hide mine.

"No it doesn't. They're just eye drops. You need to keep your eyes open."

"I'm trying to! But they hurt. Especially my left."

"I didn't say to *try* to keep them open. You need to *actually* keep them open."

As I leaned my head back for the fifth time, the doctor towered over me with eye drops in one hand and a crumpled up paper towel soaked with my tears in the other. I looked up at him. Dr. Woods had a round face and wore glasses, just like my father. Those were the only details I could make out. Between my pupils being half-dilated and the constant flow of tears, everything was blurry. Not to mention the severe inflammation in my left eye I was there for in the first place.

Dr. Woods used his fingers to pry open my

left eye, holding down my forehead with his palm. It seemed like he was using more force than necessary, though I didn't understand why *any* force was needed. I'd had eye drops put in by a different doctor – another abrasive asshole – just two days earlier. It'd taken a few tries but he got the job done without having to force my eyelids open. While Dr. Woods's stubby little fingers held open my eye, he squeezed the eye dropper just an inch above my face. And the second that first drop landed, my eyelid broke free of the doctor's fingers and slammed shut once again.

"You're being difficult. Here," Dr. Woods said, throwing the tear-soaked paper towel at me. "Dry your eyes. I'm going to send a nurse in. I'll be back when your eyes are redilated."

The doctor stormed out of the exam room, slamming the door behind him. Before it was even halfway closed, both of my middle fingers were up. With the asshole doc out of the room, I took a deep breath, put my headphones on, pressed play on my Sony Walkman, and leaned back in the exam chair.

A few minutes later, just as my watery eyes finally stopped leaking, a nurse came in. Her smile and laid-back demeanor instantly put me at ease. She was much more pleasant than the doctor, but it would've been hard not to be. It took a couple of minutes, but she managed to get the eye drops in. My sensitive blue eyes still teared up like crazy. But she got the job done and without even a hint of frustration.

Once my eyes were properly dilated, Dr. Woods came back into the room and continued the exam. He didn't say much other than the occasional order he barked at me:

"Look over there. Not there. *There.*"

"I said wide. Keep your eyes open wide."

"Stop fidgeting. You need to sit still."

The whole exam couldn't have taken more than ten minutes, but it felt like hours. Who you're in a room with plays a huge role in how fast time seems to move, almost as big a role as how physically uncomfortable you are. When you're uncomfortable *and* alone in a room with an asshole, time slows to a crawl.

As soon as he finished the exam, Dr. Woods left the room for a few minutes to go talk to my mother. She was out in the waiting room doing whatever she could to take her mind off the fact that something was seriously wrong with her son. After the doctor broke the news to her, the two of them came into the exam room to share it with me.

"You have Behcet's disease," Dr. Woods stated matter-of-factly, as if all sixteen-year-olds were supposed to know what that was.

"Finally some good news," I said. But my relief was short lived. It vanished the second I looked over at my mother. Her lip quivered as she tried to smile at me. My eyes were still dilated but her lip moved so wildly it was impossible not to notice. The doctor's face remained expressionless. "It *is* good, isn't it? Now that we know what's been causing all my symptoms, we can cure it, right?"

I glanced over at my mother again. She didn't say a word but her still-quivering lip spoke volumes.

"Right?" I asked, looking over at the doctor. "You can cure it?"

"No," Dr. Woods replied, bluntly.

"What do you mean, *no*?" I asked.

"Behcet's disease is a lifelong illness. There is no cure."

"But you can fix my eye, right?"

"The inflammation in your retina is severe," Dr. Woods explained. "It may improve slightly over time with aggressive treatment, but a full recovery is unlikely."

"What will give Ellis the best chance of recovering as much as possible?" my mother asked.

"We'll continue with the prednisone," Dr. Woods replied, turning to face my mother. "But we need to increase the dosage considerably. I'm also going to prescribe two types of eye drops. One of them is to keep your son's left eye dilated. It'll help with the pain and inflammation. The other is just more steroids.[1] But instead of taking them by mouth like the prednisone, they're eye drops. And lastly, there's one more treatment I'd strongly recommend that might make a big difference in your son's recovery. But he's not going to like it. And I'm not going to force him to do it. He's nearly an adult. He can decide for himself."

"What is it?" my mother asked leaning forward, her eyes wide.

"An intravitreal injection."

My mother leaned back in her chair. Any optimism she might've been feeling vanished. As a registered nurse, mom knew exactly what that type of injection was. She also knew how I'd react when *I* realized what it was.

"What's an in-trivial injection?" I asked.

"*Intravitreal*," Dr. Woods corrected. "It's an injection that goes deep into the eye so medicine can be delivered more closely to your retina where the

---

[1] Steroids, in this case, doesn't mean muscle-building anabolic steroids. Dr. Woods meant corticosteroids. They're used to reduce inflammation.

inflammation is."

"The doctor said it might make a big-" my mother tried to reason with me.

"Fuck that!" I yelled. "No one's sticking a needle in my eye. I'll take my chances."

"Ellis, you really should-" my mom tried again.

"No!" I replied. "Enough is enough. I'm not letting anyone stick a needle in my eye."

"Doctor," my mother pleaded with the ophthalmologist. "Can't you-"

"I'm not going to force him to do it. He can make his own decisions."

"Ellis, just think-" my mother said.

"No," I interrupted again. "No. No. No! I'm not doing it. No way. Not happening."

I wasn't going to let anyone stick a needle deep into my eye, especially a guy who'd struggled to get eye drops in there. But to Dr. Woods's credit, he earned a tiny sliver of my respect by leaving the decision up to me.[2] Hearing you're old enough to make your own decisions is music to any sixteen-year-old's ears. At that age, you're trapped between being dependent on adults and wanting to establish your own independence. Any step toward the latter is usually a welcome one. My mother, on the other hand, wholeheartedly disagreed. She thought Dr. Woods should've forced me to get the injection. But she knew better than anyone that her rebellious son wasn't going to do anything he didn't want to do.

In retrospect, I should've sucked it up and got

---

[2] Looking back, I don't think Dr. Woods had any respect for my decision making ability. He probably just didn't want to administer the shot after seeing how hard it was to just get the drops in my eyes and knew I'd refuse. Can't say I blame him.

the injection. But I let fear dominate my decision. Well, that and the fact that I was eager to get the fuck out of Mass Eye and Ear as soon as possible. If I'd gotten the injection, we would've been there a lot longer. Mom made a few more attempts at trying to convince me to do it, but I consistently refused. So we took the prescriptions Dr. Woods wrote – and more importantly my shiny, brand-new Behcet's disease diagnosis – and headed home from the city.

My mother did everything she could to hold it together. It was obvious that she wanted to burst out in tears. But being the strong, military-trained woman she was, mom didn't shed even a single drop. Not in the exam room anyway. I'm sure she fell apart as soon as we got home, though. I didn't even go in the house. After the mostly silent drive home from Boston, I needed to be alone. We pulled into our driveway, I got out of my mother's blue 1980's Dodge Caravan,[3] sparked up a Marlboro Red, and walked off down the street.

Emotions are usually pretty straightforward. *I'm incredibly angry. I'm a little afraid. I'm very happy. I'm kind of sad.* They usually come one at a time and at a certain level of intensity. But the emotions I experienced on my nicotine-fueled walk that day were anything but straightforward. On the one hand I felt extremely angry, anxious, sad, worried, defeated, disgusted, ashamed, embarrassed, and afraid. Yet I also felt slightly calm, courageous, happy, and relieved at the same time. There probably aren't many things that can fire up your limbic system like being told you have a rare, incurable, painful,

---

[3] I think it was a 1987 Dodge Grand Caravan – not that it matters at all.

lifelong illness. I certainly couldn't ever recall having such a plethora of powerful emotions floating around inside me all at once like that.

I'm sure my mother – and later my father when he got home from work and she broke the news to him – probably had a similar experience. Looking back, I really feel for what they must've went through. The only thing harder than being told that *you* are chronically ill is to be told *your child* is.

Me, my mom, my dad: we were all in shock. But now we finally had something to work with. We could finally put a name to all the strange symptoms I'd been having for years. Dr. Woods did what none of the other doctors I'd been to were able to: accurately diagnose me. Sure, he could've made at least some attempt at softening the blow when he delivered the news. He could've been nicer to me and my mom, who also thought he was an asshole (though she used a slightly-more-polite term: jerk). He could've sugarcoated the news and patiently explained what Behcet's was. But none of that mattered. Not really. It was all secondary. The only thing that truly mattered was that I finally had a diagnosis. And I had Dr. Woods to thank for it.

I was sixteen-years-old when Dr. Woods diagnosed me with Behcet's disease in 1997, though I'd been been having symptoms for years. It's hard to pinpoint exactly when – or even *what* – my first Behcet's symptom was. I can remember unexplained swelling and pain – mystery pain, as I called it when I was little – as far back as elementary school. But it was during my freshman year of high school that my body really started kicking its own ass.

"I have learned now that while those who speak about one's miseries usually hurt, those who keep silence hurt more." - C.S. Lewis

2. Little Red Bumps

High school would've been challenging enough had I been perfectly healthy. Between trying to have a social life, dealing with my parents, figuring out my rapidly changing body, and doing my actual schoolwork, I would've had my hands full. Add Behcet's disease into the mix and what would've already been challenging now becomes an unrelenting nightmare.

For the most part, freshman year sucked. Pain and embarrassment were the themes of that year. Although to be fair, they were the themes of much of my high school career. But freshman year *especially* sucked. Even my favorite class that year, band, was filled with suffering.

My first year at public high school, I played the snare drum in marching band. I'd taken lessons at a local music store from a guy I'd end up seeing at a court-mandated AA[1] meeting years later. It's funny who you run into at those things. He didn't recognize me. And I barely recognized him – at first. But it was definitely my old drum teacher. When I saw him in that church basement with a foam cup of coffee in one hand and a copy of the big book[2] in the other, a lot of things suddenly made sense. It explained why he'd often come stumbling into our lessons late. It

---

[1] Alcoholics Anonymous

[2] The "big book" is what Alcoholics Anonymous members call their handbook. It *is* a big book – but I've seen bigger.

made me understand why one week he'd be happy and cheerful, the next week he'd be withdrawn and impatient. And though I probably should've put two-and-two together a lot sooner, it explained why his breath often smelt like peppermint schnapps.

    Regardless, he was a good drummer, a good teacher, and an overall likable guy. I took lessons from him during my last two years of middle school. He taught me everything I needed to know to take band in high school freshman year. Band class was broken into two parts: the first half of the year was marching band and the second half was concert band. The second half was lots of fun. The first half totally sucked.

    Starting when I was still in middle school, I used to get these little bumps on my upper legs. They kind of looked like pimples, but not exactly. And they were freakin' everywhere. Imagine someone you've known who had terrible acne. I'm talking about someone with a faceful of red, pus-filled zits. Now picture their acne-covered face but multiply the number of pimples times ten. That's why my upper legs looked like.

    From my knees all the way to my hips, the fronts of my legs were covered with little red bumps – some not so little. Many of them had whiteheads filled with pus. Others didn't. Some of the larger bumps appeared to have smaller bumps growing out of them. It was wicked gross. And many of the bumps, when touched, hurt.

    In marching band, we used to play at all the school's football games and pep rallies. During practice, my snare drum was mounted on a stand. But when we performed, I had to wear the snare drum on a harness. Like most of the band's equipment, the harnesses were decades old. They're supposed to have a thick layer of padding on the shoulders and at the bottom where your legs hit it while marching. The padding was supposed to protect your legs not only from hitting the harness but, more importantly, from the massive screws sticking out of it. Drilled into the bottom of each harness, there were two large screws that attached to the piece of metal holding the actual drum. They went through the harness precisely where your legs hit it while marching. If the padding had still been there, it would've covered the screws. But those harnesses were so old that all of the padding had worn away years earlier.

    I would cringe just looking at one of those ancient harnesses knowing I had to put it on. As I slipped it over my head, the hard plastic harness hooked onto my bony shoulders as if it was clicking into place. The harness itself wasn't so bad. It wasn't very heavy. When I attached the snare drum – which *was* heavy – that's where the discomfort began. But it's not where it ended.

    Before every football game, the band would line up right outside of the band room. Woodwinds were in front, followed by brass instruments. Bass drum, snare drums, cymbals: we were in the back. For some reason our band teacher would have us march all the way from the band room to the football field. He'd have us start playing as soon as we began marching even though we were too far away for anyone in the stands to hear us.

    I kept my eyes focused on the sheet music clipped to my snare drum as we began marching. Left. Right. Left. Right. Every step was agony. I felt like I was being stabbed every time I took a step – because I was. The sharp screws poking through the harness jabbed me in my red-bump-covered thighs. I did everything I could to stay focused on my drumming. But in my head I was moaning and groaning with each painful step.

    Left.
Ouch, I thought.
    Right.
Ow!
    Left.
Ugh.
    Right.
Fuck!

    By the time the marching band actually got to the football field, I could feel my legs bleeding under the ultra-thin band uniform we all had to wear. While I drumrolled my way through the national anthem, blood and pus drizzled down my legs and over my knees. I eventually started wearing sweatpants under my band uniform, but even that didn't stop those screws from stabbing me.

    As the football season went on, things only got worse. Getting repeatedly stabbed in the legs by a sharp piece of metal in September when it's sixty-degrees out sucks. Getting stabbed in December when it's ten degrees *really* sucks.

    After we made our ridiculously long march out to the field, the band would sit in the the stands until it was time to perform at the halftime show. On the plus side, it gave my legs a break from literally getting screwed. But after sitting in the cold for so long, when it was time to get up at halftime, my legs hurt more than ever.

    In the stands, every once in a while we'd perform a short piece of music between plays. Or in the off chance our team actually scored a touchdown, we'd play the chorus to We Will Rock You. During those late-season games, I almost would've rather been marching around and getting stabbed in the legs than sitting in the stands. It got so cold we could barely play our instruments. Watching the cheerleaders bounce around in front of the stands provided some distraction from the cold. But it was always short lived. When you're *that* cold, it's impossible not to think about it. At least I wasn't alone. My bandmates might not have had bloody legs like me. But their noses were as Rudolph-like as mine and they couldn't feel their fingers, ears, or toes any better than I could.

"My hands feel like they're gonna fall off," Justin, a sophomore snare drummer, said.

"I know," I replied, cupping my hands around my mouth, trying to warm them with my breath. "It's fuckin' freezin' out here."

"I hope Craven lets us go in after we do the halftime show."

"Do you think he will?" I asked, sitting up a little straighter and looking over at Justin with wide eyes. "You were here last year. Did he ever let the band go in after halftime when it was this cold?"

"Yeah, *I* was here last year. But Craven wasn't. This is his first year teaching band, remember? Your guess is as good as mine."

"Oh, yeah. That's right. I forgot he's new. My guess is that we'll be here until the clock goes all the way to zero. Craven's strict like a fucking drill sergeant. I bet the old music teacher was much cooler."

"He was *cool*," Justin said. "But he didn't give a fuck about anything. Show up when you want. Leave when you want. No uniforms. We just wore whatever we wanted to the games. And he'd let us all leave right after halftime."

"I wish he was still the music teacher."

"No you don't. Mr. Craven might be a hardass, but at least he cares. At least he takes band seriously."

I can't say that Mr. Craven didn't care. But he took band a little *too* seriously if you ask me. He was fresh out of Berklee College of Music and wanted to prove himself as a music teacher. Why anyone – especially a Berklee grad – would want to be a public-high-school music teacher was beyond me. But Mr. Craven, for whatever reason, took the job and he took it very, *very* seriously.

We had to stay until the end of the game – and every other game that season. Mr. Craven insisted it would be unprofessional to leave the field before the game's end. As we sat in the stands with icy winds whipping us in the face, I remember wondering if he would've made us stay even if our noses and ears started falling off from frostbite. Justin thought then and only then, he'd let us go in. Me? I think he still would've made us stay until the end of the game.

Those little red bumps on my legs were awful. Folliculitis, which is inflammation of the hair follicle, is what the doctor diagnosed them as. They started in middle school and persisted until about halfway through my high school career. Aside from being extremely uncomfortable, those bumps caused me a lot of anxiety.

Freshman year, band was my first class of the day. Gym, which I had three days a week, was my last class. I'm not sure how or why it happened, but I ended up in a gym class full of juniors and seniors. I was the only underclassmen.

Between the ages of fourteen and eighteen, the male body changes a lot. Certain things get bigger. Some areas get hairier. If you put any male freshman in a locker room with a bunch of juniors and seniors, at least some insecurity is inevitable. But cock size and ball hair were the least of my worries. I was more concerned with being judged for my pale skin, scrawny physique, and of course my zit-covered legs.

The gym was all the way on the far side of the school. I'd power-walk down the hallway, weaving through a sea of backpack-wearing, book-carrying students so I could be one of the first to get to the locker room. I was never the very first, but I usually managed to get there before the locker room filled up. As I walked in, I'd survey the room, being extra careful what direction my eyes looked. I did my best not to make eye contact with anyone. When it happened, I'd look away immediately – any direction but down. Even more important than the no-eye-to-eye-contact rule was the no-eye-to-cock-contact rule. Getting caught looking at another guy's dick was the last thing you'd ever want to happen in a high school locker room. That's the type of thing you never live down. Nowadays I'll make *some* eye contact when I'm in the locker room at the gym. I might even nod and say hi. But I still stick to the no-eye-to-cock-contact rule. Sure, some rules are meant to be broken. But that's not one of them.

After carefully surveying the high school locker room, I'd find the most isolated spot possible. If there was an empty corner, great. The far corner away from the entrance? Even better. We didn't have assigned lockers in gym class so you could get changed wherever you wanted to. With my eyes on the floor directly in front of me, I'd rush over to my strategically chosen spot, hoping no one would try to talk to me. Fortunately, no one ever did. The upperclassmen would be too busy talking to each other about the sex they'd had the night before or the killer party they'd be going to on the weekend to have any interest in talking to me. When we played dodgeball, *that's* when they'd take an interest in me.

Facing the lockers, I'd dig through my bag and take out my sweatpants. Most of the other guys wore gym shorts, but my self-consciousness came before my physical comfort. I wouldn't have gotten changed at all if I didn't have to. With my sweatpants out and ready to go, I'd kick off my sneakers and pull down my jeans as quickly as possible. Then, as fast as lightening I'd slip on my sweatpants before anyone had a chance to see my zit-covered legs.

Those little red bumps were the first Behcet's-related skin problem I can remember having – the first of many. They caused me a lot of pain and embarrassment. Compared to what was to come, however, the bumps on my legs were nothing. At least I could hide them by wearing pants. But there'd be no hiding the avalanche of symptoms lurking right around the corner.

"You wouldn't worry so much about what others think of you if you realized how seldom they do." - Eleanor Roosevelt

3. Acne

Lots of teenagers get acne. There's nothing special about that. But the acne I'd get on my face during freshman and sophomore year was no ordinary acne. It *was* special.

The acne on my face would get so bad at times that I couldn't even bring myself to look in the mirror. When I did, I was so disgusted by what I saw that it would actually evoke a physical reaction. My stomach would feel like it was being twisted, my eyes like they were about to unleash a waterfall of tears. But *my* face wasn't the only one I couldn't look at. When my acne was bad, I found it nearly impossible to look anyone else in the eyes either. My self-esteem was so low that I had trouble looking people in the eyes to begin with. When my face was at its worst, forget it.

If you're like most people, you probably had some acne as a teen. If you're one of the lucky few who somehow managed to make it through high school without getting a single zit, fifteen-year-old me would like current me to deliver a message: "Fuck you." But few people are that lucky, so I'll assume you at least got a few zits here and there. Or maybe you had a faceful of pimples all throughout high school. Whether you only got a zit every few months or your face was usually covered in them, you know how quickly they can tank your self-esteem. A couple little zits on the forehead can send a teenager spiraling into a state of emergency faster than if they found out a nuclear missile was heading for their town. My acne was so bad that sometimes I wished an *actual* nuclear missile was heading straight for my face.

Acne almost doesn't feel like a strong-enough word for what I used to get all over my cheeks, forehead, nose, neck, and sometimes even my ears. *Nasty, painful, embarrassing pus-filled growths* is a bit more wordy, but it's also a lot more accurate. When my acne was at its worst, calling me *pizza face* would've almost seemed like a compliment. At times the acne on my face would get so bad I could actually see it. No mirrors, no reflections. I'd just look down and could see the massive pockets of pus sticking out of my face.

Cystic acne is the medical term for the big, round, sometimes-golf-ball-sized growths I'd have all over my face. When I say golf-ball sized, I'm not exaggerating. On more than one occasion during my first couple years of high school, massive cysts would grow on my forehead, nose, neck, and especially my cheeks. If I looked down, I could often see them they were so big.

Of course I tried everything I could think of to get rid of my acne or, at the very least, reduce its severity. I used Oxy Pads, but all they did was dry out my skin. Anyone who was alive in the nineties remembers Oxy Pad commercials. If the TV ads were to be believed, Oxy Pads could wipe out even the toughest acne. In reality, the only thing they wiped out was the moisture from your skin. If anything, they made my acne worse. I tried a couple different prescription creams that my pediatrician prescribed me. At the time I was still over a year away from getting diagnosed with Behcet's. None of the creams helped. Tretinoin did reduce the size of some of the whiteheads on my forehead but did nothing for the cystic acne. My doctor then prescribed me an antibiotic. Again, it made little-to-no difference.[1]

Those big red cysts didn't just come and go quickly. They slowly grew over the course of a couple weeks, then would persist for several more as they gradually shrunk. I tried to speed up the process however I could. Sometimes I made things better. Sometimes worse. Following my mother's advice, I'd press a hot, wet facecloth against my face several times a day. I'm not sure if that made things any better, but at least it didn't make things worse. What *did* sometimes make things better and sometimes worse was trying to pop them myself.

The problem was that these weren't regular zits with a whitehead on the surface. These were just big red lumps with nothing to pop. I could've squeezed them all day long and nothing ever would've come out. So I did what any desperate teenager with absolutely no medical training would've done in a pre-internet world: stick an unsterilized needle into my face. Sometimes it actually worked great. I remember one time in particular.

I was in the bathroom at my parents house equipped with a sewing needle and a facecloth. Leaning over the sink so my face was close to the mirror, I carefully lined the tip of the needle up with the center of the cyst. It was one of the worst cysts I'd ever gotten up to that point. The thing was literally

---

[1] This is a randomly placed footnote that has absolutely nothing to do with anything you've just read. I just wanted to mention that I've included a handful of footnotes in this book to either clarify something or to provide a source for certain pieces of information so you know I'm not entirely full of shit.

the size of a golf ball, stretching my skin to its limit. Slowly, I pressed the needle into my face. The cyst was so hard that my skin had no give to it. The needle went right in. And when I pulled it out, a gush of off-white pus blasted all over the bathroom mirror.

    Had I been watching anyone else perform this highly inadvisable procedure, I would've thought it was fucking gross. Even now, thinking about a younger version of myself doing it grosses me out a little bit. But at the time I remember feeling something far from disgust: satisfaction. To see that thick, not-quite-white pus splatter all over the mirror as I pressed the sides of the cyst meant my ill-conceived plan worked.

    My cyst popping didn't always go according to plan, however. One time I tried performing the same procedure on a smaller cyst. Though I can't be sure, I think I caused it to get infected. After popping the cyst and squeezing out a little bit of pus, over the course of the next couple days it grew faster than I'd ever seen one grow before. And it became a darker shade of red than any cyst I'd ever had.

    My self-esteem was already pretty low before I started getting the little red bumps on my legs. By the time the horrible cystic acne began making regular appearances on my face, forget it. I had less than zero self-esteem. I don't know if it's possible to have negative self-esteem but, if it is, I had it. I hated the way I looked and hated the way I felt. My attitude was about as healthy as my self-esteem. Negativity dominated my life at home and at school. When you're constantly suffering, it's nearly impossible to see the good in anything or anyone. Our perception of the world reflects how we feel inside. And the way I usually felt was miserable, inside and out.

When my face got really bad, I'd walk into school with my head down, unable to even make eye contact with my closest friends. All I could think about was how bad my face looked. It's hard not to think about when your acne is so bad you can see it out of the corner of your eye at all times. I'd get so paranoid that if I heard someone laughing down the hall, I'd automatically assume they were laughing at me. I thought everyone was looking at my ugly, zit-covered face all the time. It was torturous.

Looking back, the truth is very few people gave me a hard time about my acne. My friends acknowledged it at times, but didn't make fun of me because of it. I had girlfriends during those years and knew of several other female students who had crushes on me. And I now know that the other kids in high school were probably too worried about their own insecurities to be thinking about mine. I unnecessarily tortured myself worrying about what others were thinking about me for years.

Now I spend very little time worrying about the opinions others have about me. Writing a book about having sores on my balls and trying to kill myself probably wouldn't be the wisest idea if I cared what people thought. Don't get me wrong. I care very deeply about people in general, especially my friends and family. But for the most part, I don't give a fuck what any of them think about me. The way I see it, other people's opinions are none of my business – even if those opinions are about me. If they have a problem with me or the way I look, that's on *them*. It's *their* problem, not mine. And the truth is, people are so self-absorbed, so busy worrying about what everyone else is thinking about *them*, they simply don't have time to be sitting around judging *me*.

Sometime between sophomore and junior year, my pediatrician put me on a different antibiotic. It cleared up my face and the little red bumps on my legs. Over the course of just a couple months, my skin went from being covered with zits and bumps to being completely clear. But new symptoms were starting to develop in other parts of my body. And those symptoms made the little red bumps on my legs and the cystic acne on my face seem almost trivial. The level of pain and embarrassment right around the corner was far beyond anything I ever could've imagined.

> "This is your pain. This is your burning hand. It's right here. Look at it." - Tyler Durden (from Fight Club by Chuck Palahniuk)

4. Sores

If you sat down with a pen and a piece of paper trying to come up with the most painful and embarrassing illness you could, it would probably look a lot like Behcet's disease. Body parts swell up for no reason and without warning. A hundred different varieties of skin problems can happen at any time. Neurological symptoms can arise causing personality changes.

And then there are the top-two trademark symptoms of Behcet's: oral and genital ulcers.

You'd think that getting big, open, quarter-sized ulcers on your balls would be worse than getting them in your mouth – but you'd be wrong. Of all the terrible symptoms I've experienced over the years, nothing compares to the oral ulcers. Don't get me wrong: the genital ulcers were fucking painful. But the pain and suffering caused by the ones in my mouth were even worse.

For more than a decade, from my mid-teens to my mid-twenties, I always had at least a couple ulcers in my mouth and on my balls. If you've ever had a canker sore, you know how much they hurt. Behcet's sores are like canker sores times a hundred. They're bigger, more painful, and last longer.

When I was a kid, I used to get canker sores every once in a while. My mother got them, too. She told me hers were usually caused or worsened by excessive salt intake. Mine didn't seem to be. They'd come and go with no rhyme or reason. I could eat half a bag of potato chips and be fine. Mom, she'd get canker sores if she had more than a few chips. I also got strep throat a lot as a child. From what I've read, that's common for a lot of people with Behcet's.[1]

The ulcers really started getting bad around the middle of high school. After the antibiotics cleared up my face and legs, I enjoyed a short period of time where my skin was perfectly clear, head to toe. It was during that brief asymptomatic window that I had sex for the first time. You probably don't need to know that. But since I'm already talking about my balls in this chapter, I figured I'd throw it in.

During the few months that I didn't seem to have any Behcet's-related symptoms, I had a girlfriend named Heather. We met when I was working at McDonald's. She liked my long, dyed-black hair and slipped me a carefully-folded note to let me know. That's how it was done back in the nineties. There were no friend requests or PMs. No emails or DMs. If you liked someone, you'd write them a letter and then fold it with surgical precision to get it just right. There was a real art to it.

I thought Heather was cute and we started seeing each other. Before long, we were having sex in her bed – and in her mother's bed, her brother's bed, the floor, the couch, the McDonald's bathroom, and every other place we found ourselves alone. Heather took my virginity but, to this day, she still doesn't know. I didn't exactly lie to her, but I didn't tell her the truth either. Maybe someday I will. I'm sure she'll get a kick out of it. Though I haven't seen her in close

---

[1] Colucci, R., D'Erme, A., Moretti, S., & Lotti, T. (2012). Potential infectious etiology of Behcet's disease. *Pathology Research International.* Retrieved November 3, 2020 from https://www.hindawi.com/journals/pri/2012/595380

to two decades, we're friends on Facebook.

Heather and I only lasted for two-or-three months before we broke up. It was around that time the genital ulcers started. I'd already been getting the ones in my mouth off and on for years. Although I didn't know it at the time, I was only a couple months away from getting the inflammation in my left eye that would lead to my diagnosis. Had I not started getting the genital ulcers when I did, Dr. Woods might not have been able to properly diagnose me. He knew that oral and genital ulcers were common Behcet's symptoms. Between the ulcers, skin problems, inflammation in my eye, and some other symptoms, he made the diagnosis with confidence.

The open sores on my balls hurt. They hurt a lot. But the ones in my mouth were even worse. It hurt to eat. It hurt to talk. It hurt to brush my teeth. Naturally, I started doing very little of each. It even hurt to breath through my mouth when the sores were really bad. The only foods I could eat without being in pain were things like yogurt or mac and cheese. I wish there was a way to know how many boxes of Kraft macaroni and cheese I've put down over the years. It must be in the thousands. Most people probably would've gotten sick of it a long time ago, but I could eat a box right now. The people at Kraft are doing something right because I just can't seem to get enough.

Brushing my teeth was agonizing. Sometimes the oral ulcers would be on my gums, sometimes my tongue, and sometimes the insides of my cheeks – often all three. I did my best to brush around them but, when they filled up half of my mouth, it was nearly impossible. When the bristles of my toothbrush hit an open sore, the sharp, stabbing pain would vibrate throughout my entire head. I started brushing so delicately that my teeth rarely got properly cleaned. Sometimes when I really had a lot of mouth ulcers, I wouldn't brush at all. The pain was simply unbearable. Between the damage caused by the inflammation in my gums and my light-handed brushing technique, by my late teens I started having a lot of dental problems. Though generally not considered one of the main symptom of Behcet's disease, dental problems are common in people with the diagnosis.[1]

When I had a lot of oral ulcers, it even hurt to talk. I'd always been an introvert, but the sores in my mouth made me talk even less. Instead of saying hello, I'd nod and wave. If the answer to a question was a low number, I'd communicate it with my fingers instead of my voice. Instead of saying "I don't know," I'd shrug my shoulders. In class, I'd slump down at my desk to avoid eye contact with the teachers, trying to doing whatever I could to not get called on. I went to great lengths to keep my mouth shut because sometimes talking hurt so badly it made my eyes water.

But enough about my mouth. Let's talk about my balls. Shortly after Heather and I broke up, I started to get sores on my scrotum just like the ones in my mouth. I know *scrotum* is a medical term, but it sounds so much dirtier to me than *balls* for some reason. Anyway, I started getting genital lesions and they weren't too bad at first. To be honest, when I first started getting them I thought they were just another strange part of puberty that no one talked about. I

---

[1] Mumcu, G., Ergun, T., Inanc, N., Fresko, I., et al. (2004). Oral health is impaired in Behcet's disease and is associated with disease severity. *Rheumatology*, 43(8):1028-33.

certainly didn't want to talk about them. But as time went on, they got progressively worse.

The first sores on my balls were small. They were little ulcers, each about the size of a ladybug. None of them hurt too badly and they went away after about a week. And once they were gone, it was as if they were never there. No marks. No scars. Nothing. But before long the ulcers started getting worse. They got bigger in size and stuck around longer. Dime-sized sores would appear on my balls and linger for weeks. Those often *did* leave scars and they hurt like hell.

The dime-sized ulcers on my balls would come and go for the better part of the next decade. Just as the ones in my mouth often made it hurt to talk, the ones on my balls often made it hurt to walk. They'd even wake me up in the middle of the night whenever I shifted my body. And worst of all, when the genital ulcers were really bad, they'd interfere with one of my favorite adolescent pastimes: masturbation. Even though I never got any sores on the shaft or head of my penis, tugging away at it would jiggle my balls. And when I had sores on them, it really hurt. Sometimes a lot. But it never stopped me from rubbing one out when I was alone and in the mood – which was pretty much always.

As if getting dime-sized ulcers on my balls all the time wasn't enough, every so often I'd get an even-bigger one. There were a few that were so bad I still remember them to this day. It's hard to forget something that left a quarter-sized scar on your balls. A quarter is worth two-and-a-half times what a dime is worth and weighs about two-and-a-half times more. But a quarter-sized ulcer on your genitals doesn't hurt two-and-a-half times more than a dime-sized one: it hurts a-hundred-times more.

There were two ulcers that still shoot a chill down my spine and right to my crotch whenever I think about them. One was on the right side of my balls, the other on my left. That one was the worst genital ulcer I ever got. On the left side of my balls and in the worst-possible spot, I had a big, open, quarter-sized ulcer that lingered for months. It was in the exact spot my balls would rub against my leg as I walked. Every step was agony. It reminded me of the sharp screws that would jab into the little red bumps on my legs during marching band a couple years earlier. But this was worse. Way worse.

Every movement, no matter how slight, hurt – some more than others. Moving around at home wasn't so bad because I could hold my balls while I walked. But unless you're doing a Michael Jackson impression, grabbing your balls in public is generally frowned upon.[1] So I had no choice but to suck it up and deal with the pain whenever I had somewhere to be. I was far too embarrassed to tell anyone about the genital ulcers and suffered silently through each excruciating day.

Showering was a nightmare. The water would sting like dozens of angry wasps – and I just happened to know what that felt like. When I was little, maybe five or six, I ran right into a wasp's nest while playing outside. My mother counted over two-dozen stings all over my body as she tried to ease her screaming son's pain. That was not a fun day. But on the bright side, I've had absolutely no fear of bees or wasps ever since: the silver lining of getting stung by

---

[1] If you've never seen MJ dance, one of his signature moves was the crotch-grab.

dozens of wasps as a child. To this day, if a bee or a wasp gets in the house, I'll walk right up to it and kill it with my bare hand.

Now back to the water stinging the quarter-sized ulcer on my balls. Hot, cold, lukewarm: the temperature didn't matter. I had to wash my balls with such precision you'd think I was putting together a model airplane or doing brain surgery down there. I'd carefully try to navigate around the massive ulcer, doing my best not to touch it. Sometimes I'd hit it by accident. The pain was so intense my knees would slam together and a string of obscenities would flow from my also-ulcer-filled mouth.

"Motherfucking son of a goddamn... Fuck, that hurt!"

When it came to cleaning the actual ulcer itself, I had to psych myself up first. I figured that the cleaner I kept it, the faster it would heal. So the last thing I did in the shower was lightly drag a soapy facecloth over the deep, quarter-sized ulcer.

"This is going to sting like a motherfucker," I told myself. "But it's necessary. It's only going to hurt for a minute. Just do it and get it over with."

Gently, I'd wash the wide-open ulcer on the left side of my balls.

"Fuuuuuuuuuck!"

Genital and oral ulcers are two of Behcet's trademark symptoms. Both painful, both embarrassing. And Behcet's is an equal-opportunity embarrasser and pain bringer. It doesn't discriminate based on sex. Women with Behcet's obviously don't get ulcers on their balls: they get them mostly on their vulvas, but also inside their vaginas.[2] While genital

---

[2] Senusi, A., Seoudi, N., Bergmeier, L., & Fortune, F.

and oral ulcers are two of Behcet's most-common symptoms, they certainly aren't the only ones. It wouldn't be long before I'd learn that firsthand by getting hit with a new wave of strange symptoms – a wave of symptoms that would eventually lead to getting diagnosed.

(2015). Genital ulcer severity score and genital health quality of life in Behcet's disease. *Orphanet Journal of Rare Diseases*, 10, 117.

"Pain is inevitable. Suffering is not." - M. Kathleen Casey

5. Knee Surgery

Sweet sixteen. Oh, what a year.
I can't say it was *all* bad. A few good things happened to me that year. For one, I lost my virginity. That definitely goes in the sweet column. I also got my driver's license as soon as I turned sixteen-and-a-half. More sweetness. And right when I was legally old enough to work, I got my first real job at McDonald's. We'll call that one sweet and sour like the popular McNugget dipping sauce.

Don't get me wrong: it was mostly sweet. In fact, in a lot of ways working at McDonald's was fucking awesome. I doubt there are many Mickey D's employees out there who would refer to their job as *fucking awesome*. But for me and my friends, it most definitely was.

There weren't any McDonald's in the town where I grew up, but there was one just over the border in a neighboring town. The store manager, Diana, was the mother of a good friend of mine. Not only did she hire me, she hired her son and close to a dozen of our friends. Every shift we had a blast. But it wasn't like we just sat around slacking off the whole time. We were all hard workers (okay, maybe not *all*, but most) and got everything done that we needed to. But we always had a freakin' blast doing it.

I'd been working at McDonald's for about nine months when Heather and I broke up. Shortly after the breakup, I started having some stiffness in my right knee. I didn't think anything of it at first. Just one more mysterious symptom to add to the list. My knee didn't hurt, so I saw no reason to do anything about it. I figured it would eventually go away on its own like most of the other strange symptoms I'd experienced over the years.

But it didn't. It did the exact opposite: it got much worse.

Every day my right knee got a little bit bigger and a little bit stiffer. During the next seven-to-ten days, my knee went from being slightly stiff to completely unable to move. It was almost as if I didn't have a knee at all. Just one long bone going from my hip to my foot. Over the course of just a little more than a week, I went from my knee being able to bend its normal hundred-and-eighty-or-so degrees to only being able to bend maybe five degrees, if that.

The stiffness wasn't the only thing getting worse. Every morning when I woke up, the swelling in my right knee would be worse than the day before. Each day it took on the size of a new fruit. At first it was just a little bump: a blueberry. Then it got a little bigger: a raspberry. The next day my knee was as swollen as a medium-sized strawberry. After that, a plum. Then a peach. At this point, I could only bend my knee about halfway. But the swelling continued. The next day it grew to the size of your average wild, non-genetically-modified apple. Day after that it was as big as a GMO[1] orange like the ones you find at Walmart and most grocery stores. But my knee didn't stop there. At this point I could only bend it about forty-five degrees. But the swelling continued. The next morning my knee was as big as a pear. A day or two later, it'd grown to the size of a grapefruit – a big,

---

[1]   Genetically modified organisms (GMOs). GMO fruit is generally bigger, sweeter, and grows faster than non-GMO fruit.

round, GMO grapefruit. Now I couldn't even bend my leg by a single inch.

Surprisingly, my right knee didn't start to hurt very much until it reached the grapefruit stage. It *would* hurt when I tried to bend it too far from about the plum stage onward. But if I was just sitting or standing with my leg straight, it didn't really hurt. One one level, that's a good thing. Nobody likes to be in pain. But on another level, that lack of pain prevented me from seeking help until I couldn't move my leg at all.

My knee only hurts when I bend it, I reasoned. *So as long as I don't bend it, I'm all good. I mean, yeah, it probably shouldn't be swelling up like a balloon. At this rate my knee will be the size of a watermelon by the end of the month. But my weird-ass body has been doing shit like this to me for years and it almost always goes back to normal on its own... eventually. I'm sure the swelling in my knee will start to go down soon.*

It didn't.

It only got worse until I was hobbling around with one normal leg and one as stiff as a board. I couldn't run. I couldn't ride my bike. I couldn't skateboard. And I certainly couldn't hide it anymore. My parents noticed me hobbling around the house and insisted on a show and tell session. Reluctantly, I showed them my knee and told them about how it'd been getting more and more swollen with each passing day. My mother took me to my pediatrician and he referred me to an orthopedic surgeon at nearby Morton Hospital.

"You're *sure* there was no trauma?" the surgeon asked for the third time. "You didn't fall down a flight of stairs? Or recently get into a car accident?"

"For the ten-thousandth time, no," I replied.

"Alright, I believe you," he lied.

The surgeon pulled the largest syringe I'd ever seen out of a drawer. Then he reached into the drawer next to it and pulled out the largest needle I'd ever seen. He attached the needle to the syringe and rolled over to me in his wheeled stool. I knew exactly what he was about to do with it.

"Is that going in my-"

"Unfortunately," the surgeon replied, "it is. We need to drain as much of that fluid out as possible."

After sterilizing my knee, the surgeon plunged the long needle into the grapefruit-sized lump growing out of it. He slowly pulled back the plunger and the syringe started filling up with yellowish-green pus. I still remember being shocked by the brightness of the color. It was practically neon and looked like it might've glowed in the dark had one of us flipped the exam-room light switch off. The doctor sucked out an entire syringe of that yellow-green slime and emptied it into a bucket. It barely made a dent in the lump on my knee. He went in again and sucked out another full syringe of pus. Then another. It cut the size of the lump down by more than half, but I still could barely bend my knee.

"Unfortunately, I'm going to need to get in there," the surgeon said. I really didn't like how many times he'd used the word *unfortunately*. "I need to look around to see if I can figure out a cause and clean out the rest of the pus."

"Like, surgery?" I asked.

"Not *like* surgery. Surgery. Unfortunately, there's no other way for me to get in there and see what's going on. But don't worry. It's a simple procedure. I've done hundreds of them. Although, I've never seen such severe inflammation with no signs of any trauma."

On June 16, 1997, a few days after my initial consult with the surgeon, I'd be back at Morton to have arthroscopic surgery. Lying in a hospital bed surrounded by doctors, I counted backward from a hundred until I lost consciousness. I made it to about eighty-five before the drugs knocked me out. When I came to who-knows-how-long later, my right knee was wrapped in coban[1] with a small tube coming out of it. The tube was attached to a round plastic reservoir to collect any remaining fluid that might come out of my knee.

When I first woke up, I still had enough of whatever sedatives the anesthesiologist pumped me full of floating around in my system that I could barely feel my knee – or anything for that matter. But as the drugs wore off, I became more and more aware of how strange my right knee felt. It wasn't from the surgery itself, though. My knee felt strange because I had a tube going about six-inches deep into it.

They let me leave Morton a couple hours after I woke up. Though I could leave the hospital, the irrigation tube couldn't leave my knee for several days. I had to walk around with that thing everywhere I went. Fortunately, I didn't have anywhere to go other than to the fridge, the bathroom, and my bedroom. The one good thing to come out of all this was that I got to stay home from school for a few days.

---

[1] Short for cohesive bandage. It's a type of medical wrap that sticks to itself, making it easy to stay in place.

I spent most of the week on the couch watching TV while my parents were at work and my fellow classmates were in school. All throughout middle-and-high school, just about every time I stayed home sick from school, I watched The Hobbit. I'm not talking about the unnecessarily long three-part piece of shit Peter Jackson put out in the 2010s. I'm talking about the seventy-eight-minute animated version of The Hobbit that came out in 1977. I had a copy of a copy of it on VHS[1] and I watched it every time I stayed home sick from school. I guess you could call it my comfort movie. I watched it several times in the days following my surgery.

It was during this mini-vacation that I had my first experience with opioids – the first of many. The surgeon prescribed me some Tylenol #3s[2] to take every few hours for the pain. The label said to take one-to-two tablets every four-to-six hours. One tablet did nothing for my knee pain. But *two* tabs not only made my knee feel a little better, they made *me* feel better. Like, *a lot* better. Those pills made the nearly constant depression and anxiety I felt disappear entirely – for a few hours, at least. It was nice, something I definitely wanted more of.

The Tylenol #3s even helped ease the pain of my oral and genital ulcers. They didn't kill the pain entirely, but reduced it enough that I could eat

---

[1] Back before Netflix or even DVDs, there was VHS (Video Home System). If you don't know what VHS tapes were, they we big cassettes us old people used to play and record videos. VHS became popular in the early 1970s and stopped being produced in 2008.

[2] Tylenol #3s contain 300 milligrams (mg) of acetaminophen and 30 mg of codeine, a natural opiate found in the opium poppy.

comfortably. I remember tearing through the kitchen while home from school, stuffing my face with all the things that were usually too painful to eat. And after wolfing down handfuls of pretzels, peanuts, and whatever else I could find, I'd limp out onto the porch and fire up a Marlboro Red.

Cigarettes, to a smoker, taste good. To a smoker who's on opioids, cigarettes taste like fucking heaven. It took me a couple days to figure out why my Marlboros tasted so good all of a sudden, but I eventually realized it was because of the Tylenol #3s. Opioids and nicotine go together like peanut butter and jelly. Add some caffeine into the mix and you've got a winning combo.

I always enjoyed smoking cigarettes. The first of the day was usually the best, but they were all good. I had my first cigarette at the age of ten. By the time I was in my mid-teens, I'd be smoking a half-pack a day at least. Sometimes I'd go through a full pack or more. Obviously, I smoked to get my nicotine fix. The fact that it was rebellious and cool made me like smoking even more. But cigarettes had another effect that I loved: they made my mouth ulcers feel better. You'd think that sucking in smoke would make them feel worse. But sure enough, cigarettes would greatly reduce the pain in my mouth while I was smoking them and for a few minutes afterward. I mentioned it to one of my doctors a few years later and he confirmed it: smoking can reduce the pain associated with oral ulcers. He didn't give me the smoking endorsement I'd hoped for and told me I should still try to quit. But at least I knew I wasn't crazy. They really did help the pain.

After a few days of hanging around the house doing nothing but slacking off, snacking off, and jacking off, I went back to the orthopedic surgeon to get the tube removed from my knee. I figured there'd be some lengthy removal procedure, but I was wrong. He just yanked the thing out. I remember being surprised by how deep into my knee it went. That tube went a good six inches into me. It felt incredibly strange having it pulled out, but didn't really hurt. And it was over in a second.

    The doctor said I could go back to school. I still needed crutches to get around, but my knee was slowly getting better. On my first day back, everyone asked me what happened to my knee. I really didn't know how to explain it to them. I didn't understand it myself. So I did what I thought was best at the time: I lied.

    "Dude, what'd you do to your leg?" a friend asked as I limped into school.

    "Nothing, really," I replied, doing my best not to make eye contact.

    "Bullshit! You're on crutches. And your knee is all wrapped up. Something must've happened."

    "Skateboarding accident," I explained, casually.

    "What happened?" my friend asked with intense interest.

    "I was trying to grind down a railing and fell. Busted my knee up."

    "Damn, that's crazy! Where'd it happen?"

    "Boston," I answered confidently, almost as if I believed it myself.

    "They give you any good drugs?"

    "Fuck yeah they did. I've been high as a kite for days."

    "Awesome!" my friend yelled, high-fiving me in the hallway.

That wasn't the first time I lied about one of my strange symptoms and it wouldn't be the last. I had no idea how to explain the things that kept happening to me. My pediatrician and other doctors I'd been to couldn't even explain them. It was terrifying. I had no idea why my body kept attacking itself and neither did anyone else. Little did I know that, within a week, I'd meet a doctor named Scott Woods who'd be able to explain everything.

"When pain brings you down, don't be silly, don't close your eyes and cry, you just might be in the best position to see the sun shine." - Alanis Morissette

6. Retinitis

Just five days after having knee surgery, my body decided to throw some more suffering at me. I guess skin problems, sores in my mouth and on my balls, and an inflamed knee wasn't enough. It wanted me to really see how powerfully it could fuck my world up. And it did so by blinding me. I woke up that Saturday morning with intense pain in my left eye, my vision so blurry that I couldn't see.

The night before I'd stayed up late to watch TV, jerk off, and chain smoke Marlboro Reds out my bedroom window. It was a typical night and nothing seemed out of the ordinary. If something was wrong with my vision, I'm sure I would've noticed it while flipping through the Barely Legal magazine I'd "read" a hundred times before. But when I woke up the next morning, I felt like a pissed-off wasp flew into my pupil and stung me in the back of the eye twenty-eight times.[1] There's sharp pain and then there's *sharp* pain. I'd never experienced anything like it before and I haven't since.

This is one of the scariest aspects of having Behcet's disease: how quickly the symptoms can come out of nowhere. With no warning at all, you can lose your vision, hearing, mobility, or even your life in a matter of hours, minutes, or even seconds. I went

---

[1] Why twenty-eight? Because I know what it feels like to get stung by twenty-eight wasps at the same time. That's how many distinct puncture wounds my mother counted after I'd run into the wasps' nest when I was little.

from having perfect eyesight to being blind in my left eye overnight – *literally* overnight. There were no warning signs or other indications that something terrible was about to happen. It just happened.

Immediately after waking, I ran upstairs and told my mother about the pain in my eye and loss of vision. Even though there was nothing observably wrong with my eye, she could tell how serious it was by the way I acted. The fact that I told her anything at all spoke volumes. I usually kept all the strange symptoms I'd had over the years to myself as best as I could. Very rarely did I vocalize being unhappy or in pain. So when I did, she listened.

My mother immediately got on the phone to get me an appointment with an ophthalmologist. During the week, it wouldn't have been much of a problem. But it was a Saturday morning and most ophthalmologists were out playing golf, spending time with their families and mistresses, sleeping off a hangover from their Friday-night-drinking binge, or doing whatever it is they do in their free time. In the case of the on-call ophthalmologist who reluctantly agreed to come in on his day off to see me, he was gardening. And he made it clear the whole time we were together that he would've rather been in his garden than examining some rebellious, long-haired sixteen-year-old punk's eye.

Of all the medical and dental emergencies I've had over the years, the serious ones always seem to happen on the weekend. You'd think that since there are two-and-a-half-times-more days during the week than there are on the weekend, most emergencies would fall during the week. But for some reason that never seems to be the case. Friday evening to Sunday night seems to be my body's prime time for causing trouble. If I didn't know any better, I'd think that Behcet's goes out of its way to not only be the most embarrassing and painful illness it can possibly be, but also the most inconvenient.

Dr. Masterson was the small-town ophthalmologist who my mother took me to see. His attitude was unpleasant to say the least. He set the rudeness bar pretty high that Saturday morning, but Dr. Woods would top it a couple days later. Those big city doctors have to be better at everything.

Like Dr. Woods, Dr. Masterson wore glasses. Maybe eye doctors choose their specialty out of some hidden insecurity about their own less-than-perfect eyesight. Perhaps it makes them feel better about themselves to point out problems with other people's eyes. Or maybe it's just a coincidence.

After dilating both of my eyes, the doctor used several intimidating pieces of equipment to examine them. I'd never had anything more than the routine eye exam that came with my yearly physical or the half-assed eye-and-ear exams they did in school. So everything was new to me. I remember being interested in all the cool medical equipment, but mostly just feeling scared and uncomfortable.

My light-blue eyes are really sensitive and always have been. Sensitive to light, sensitive to touch – just sensitive in general. I guess that's the price to be paid for having pretty blue eyes. The doctor got frustrated with me because they kept watering and he had trouble administering the various types of eye drops. But he eventually got my eyes dilated and started the exam. It was awkward. As the doctor peered into my eyes, he shined a light in them bright enough to pierce my soul. But it was one particular part of the exam that really made my heart rate skyrocket. The doctor put even more eye drops in and had me rest my chin on a small piece of padding. He slowly pulled over a piece of equipment that looked like a small cone and lined it up with my left eye.

"That's not going to touch or go in my eye, is it?" I asked, practically shaking.

"No," the doctor lied. "It's not."

"And it's not going to hurt, right?"

"You won't feel a thing," he lied again.

My heart started beating faster and faster as the tip of the cone got closer and closer. My left eye was too blurry to see it approaching, but I could see it out of the corner of my right. The strange cone touched my eyeball and a strong puff of air came out of the tip. Though it didn't exactly hurt, it was extremely uncomfortable. It felt like someone took a tiny straw, stuck one end in my eye, and blew on the other. The doctor then repeated the process with my right eye. That was even worse because, this time, I could see it coming. The cone went right into my eye and I felt a blast of air inside my pupil. It felt *really* strange.

The whole time, the doctor made no attempt at hiding his resentment for having to come in on his day off. It almost made me feel guilty for having an inflamed eyeball on a non-weekday. But he also made no attempt to hide how serious my condition was. And that made me feel even worse.

"I've never seen anything like it," Dr. Masterson said.

Not exactly something you want to hear come out of a doctor's mouth. That was the *second* time I'd heard a doctor say it that month. The surgeon I'd seen said something similar about the inflammation in my knee. I can't tell you how many times I've heard some variation of that phrase over the years. Besides Dr. Masterson, I can recall hearing it from a radiologist, an internist, two dermatologists, and an orthopedic surgeon – and that's just off the top of my head. Nowadays I take a certain pride in hearing a doctor tell me they've never seen such severe inflammation. But back then it was just scary.

"What do you mean you've never seen anything like it?" I asked. "You're an eye doctor."

"I'm a small-town ophthalmologist," Dr. Masterson explained. "I've never seen inflammation this severe come on so quickly."

"But you can fix it, right?" I asked. "Do you know what's causing it, at least?"

"I don't know. And no. I have no idea."

Nothing that came out of Dr. Masterson's mouth that morning made me feel better. His official diagnosis was severe uveitis and retinitis of unknown origin. I left his office feeling worse than when I'd come in. I'm sure my mother felt the same way. When her and I left the office, we went to the pharmacy to fill the eye-drop prescriptions he'd written me. While the meds were no doubt useful, it was something else the doctor gave me that turned out to be invaluable. No, I'm not talking about the bill for seeing a specialist on a Saturday. That had a highly-inflated-but-finite price. I'm talking about the referral he gave me to see a retina specialist in Boston named Dr. Scott Woods.

That pompous ophthalmologist – or pomphthalmologist as I would've called him had I thought of it twenty-four years ago instead of just now – managed to do something for me that no other doctor had been able to. Before going into Boston to see Dr. Woods at Mass Eye and Ear, I'd already been to five or six different local doctors for various ailments. None of them had any idea what was wrong with me. They just did what doctors typically do: try to patch up whatever symptom I was there for and send me on my way. But Dr. Woods did something for me that was much more valuable, something that would change my life forever – he gave me the name of what had been wreaking havoc on my life for years.

    Most people probably wouldn't be thrilled to find out they have a chronic illness. But after all the strange, painful, and embarrassing symptoms I'd been having, it was nice to finally know what was causing them. Putting a name to my suffering legitimized it in a way. Getting diagnosed with Behcet's disease eased the anxiety of not knowing what was wrong with me. Yet at the same time, it added the anxiety of knowing I'd have to deal with this shitty illness for the rest of my life. But at least it now had a name. At least I knew that there were other people out there suffering like me.

    When you're going through something difficult and you feel like you're the only one on the planet going through it, it makes dealing with it even harder. It adds an element of loneliness on top of all the other complex emotions swirling through your head. But knowing that there were other people out there dealing with the same illness made me feel a tiny bit better. And it made my parents feel a lot better.

    My mom and dad were both registered nurses with impressive resumes. They'd both served in the military, each being honorably discharged as captains. Before I was born, my mother had worked at Mass

General, one of the most prestigious hospitals in the country. And my father went on to graduate school to become a clinical nurse specialist. Still, all the training and experience in the world doesn't prepare you to deal with your own sick child. Not knowing what was wrong with their son made them feel helpless. They didn't know what to do and the doctors I'd been to didn't have any useful advice for them. When I was finally diagnosed, it gave them something to work with. They no longer felt *totally* helpless. It allowed them to do *something*.

      That something was education. They read books about Behcet's disease, scouring local libraries in a pre-internet world for the few existing titles about the disorder. They researched different medications used to treat the disease. They even attended a conference of the American Behcet's Disease Association, conveniently held in Boston the year I was diagnosed. They learned all that they could about their son's illness. But when they tried to educate me, I didn't want to hear even a single word of it.

"You will know the truth and the truth will set you free." - John 8:32

7. Denial

I was sixteen-years old when I got diagnosed with Behcet's disease. At the time, all I cared about was playing guitar, hanging out with friends, skateboarding, and chasing girls. Well, that and masturbating when the chasing girls thing wasn't going so well. But the last thing I wanted to do was learn about Behcet's disease.

As much of a relief as it was to know what had been causing all my strange symptoms, I didn't want to believe it. I didn't want to accept that I had a lifelong illness that would fuck my life up in ways I couldn't possibly imagine. I *couldn't* accept it. Even though the diagnosis fit my symptoms perfectly, I refused to believe I had Behcet's. As it turned out, I was suffering from another ailment: ostrich syndrome (though I was never formally diagnosed). I thought if I buried my head in the sand, if I ignored the mountain of evidence pointing to Behcet's, it would eventually go away.

Well, it didn't.

My body continued to attack itself. And I continued to pretend like nothing was wrong, which wasn't easy. It's hard to ignore something when reminders are everywhere; when you have to take a handful of pills first thing in the morning and the last thing at night; when you look in the mirror and one of your pupils is twice the size of the other; when you're hobbling around on crutches everywhere you go cause your knee won't bend; when people you've known your whole life start treating you differently;

when you have several doctor's appointments every week; when you have literature about Behcet's from two concerned parents all over the house; and when you feel like shit from the moment you wake up until the moment you go to bed everyday. Still, in spite of all this, I refused to accept that I had Behcet's disease.

You've probably heard of the five stages of grief. When most people think of them, they think about the death of a loved one. But these stages can happen not only when you lose a loved one, but also when you lose anything you care about. They should be called the five stages of loss, really.[1] Getting diagnosed with a chronic illness is a lot like losing someone close to you. The only difference is that you're not losing someone else – you're losing *yourself*. You're losing the life that you pictured yourself living. When you're in mourning, it's not the deceased you're mourning – not exactly. It's the loss of the future you planned to have with the deceased. You're mourning the loss of all the memories you were expecting to make with them. The same is true when you're diagnosed with a lifelong disease. You mourn the loss of the healthy life you were planning on living.

The first of the five stages of grief is denial, followed by anger, bargaining, depression, and acceptance. Though many psychologists criticize the five stage model,[2] I can tell you that I absolutely experienced all of them after being diagnosed. Maybe

[1] Originally developed by psychiatrist Elisabeth Kübler-Ross, the five stages of grief were originally meant to describe the process terminally ill patients go through after being diagnosed and not the death of a loved one.

[2] Stroebe, M., Schut, H., & Boerner, K. (2017). Cautioning health-care professionals. *Omega*, 74(4):455-473.

not in that exact order, but denial was definitely first and acceptance last.

It would be years before I truly accepted that I had Behcet's. But not only did I refuse to believe it myself, I did my best to hide it from everyone in my life: friends, girlfriends, classmates, and coworkers. Only my closest friends and family knew that I'd been diagnosed. And even then I had a hard time being honest with them. Sometimes I'd flat out lie to protect my embarrassing secret. I thought that if people knew I had an illness, they'd think I was weak. So I made stuff up.

Dr. Woods put me on even more prednisone and eye drops. Those big twenty-milligram prednisone tablets were fucking nasty. I had to take three a day for months. Even to this day, I can remember the bitter aftertaste they'd leave in my mouth. Back then I wasn't the experienced pill popper I am today. Now I can swallow a handful of pills like it's nothing. But at the age of sixteen, I hadn't yet mastered the pop, pour, tilt, swallow method. Sometimes it would take me up to three sips of water to get the prednisone down, which was two too many. If those nasty little pills sat on my tongue for more than a second, their disgusting taste would would soak into it and linger for up to fifteen minutes. It was fucking awful.

In addition to the prednisone pills, Dr. Woods also put me on two types of eye drops. One of them was prednisolone, a corticosteroid very similar to prednisone. The other eye drops, though I've since forgotten the name, were used to keep my left eye dilated at all times. I hated them. I hated all of it, the pills *and* the eye drops. But I especially hated the eye drops. It was bad enough needing to have them put in when I went to the ophthalmologist. Having to put them in myself every single morning was awful.

But the eye drops themselves were only half of the reason why I couldn't stand them. The other half? Because they made me look like a freak. There I was, already limping around the halls of my high school on crutches. Now I had one normal-looking eye and one that looked like I'd just eaten a handful of psychedelic mushrooms.[1] My right eye appeared as if nothing was out of the ordinary – because it wasn't. If anything, my right pupil was a little smaller than normal. Codeine and other opioids cause your pupils to constrict. So my right one might've been extra small from the Tylenol #3s I was still taking. But my left pupil was widely dilated. By comparison, it was several times larger than my right. Anyone who looked me in the eyes noticed right away.

"Dude, your eye!" a friend noticed the second I hobbled into school for the first time since being diagnosed. "The fuck happened to it?"

"Oh, it's nothing really," I replied, desperately trying not to make eye contact with him or anyone else.

"Get the fuck out of here, man. One week you come limping into school on crutches. The next week one of your eyes is twice the size of the other one. Something's up."

"You really want to know the truth?" I asked, scrambling to come up with some sort of plausible explanation.

"Uh, yeah."

"I busted up my knee skateboarding in Boston

---

[1] Shrooms, LSD, and many other hallucinogens make your pupils dilate (widen). Opioids do the opposite. They make them constrict.

a couple weeks ago. When I fell, I whacked my head on the pavement so hard that it ruptured something in my left eye. So I have to use these stupid eye drops to keep it dilated so it can heal."

"That's so fucking cool!" my friend replied. "Do you have the eye drops with you?"

"Why?" I asked.

"Cause I want to use 'em. Your eyes look badass. Straight up freaky. It's awesome. I want one big eye and one normal eye, too."

"Sorry, man. I have to keep them at home."

"Oh well," he said. My friend turned away and began yelling at the top of his lungs, "Hey everyone. Check out Ellis's eyes. They're super freaky!"

Skateboarding was my go-to excuse for many of the strange things that happened to me. Everyone knew I liked to skate and that injuries were commonplace among skateboarders. None of my classmates questioned my ridiculous explanations. I have no idea if they actually believed them or not. Bu they all seemed to.

I've never been comfortable lying. It certainly seems to come naturally for a lot of people, but I'm not one of them and never have been. However, the embarrassment of people knowing I had a rare disease outweighed my dislike for lying. And even if I had been comfortable telling the truth about my recently diagnosed illness, I'm not sure I would've been able to. If I'd tried, the above conversation might've gone something like this:

"Dude, your eye. The fuck happened to it?" my friend asked.

"Nothing," I replied.

"Bullshit! You must've done *something* to it."

"No. I really didn't."
"Then why is one twice the size of the other."
"Eye drops."
"You can buy eye drops that make you look all freaky deaky? Awesome. Where can I get some?"
"I think you can only get them from a doctor."
"So how did *you* get them?"
"From my doctor."
"But how? For what?"
"I don't know. My eye hurt and my vision was blurry so he gave me the eye drops."
"What caused the blurriness and pain?"
"Behcet's disease, I think."
"What's that?"
"I'm not really sure, to be honest."

Even after being diagnosed with Behcet's, I still didn't know how to explain it in a way that made sense. I didn't *want* to know how to explain it. I just wanted the lousy thing to go away and never come back. The thought of my classmates, teachers, friends, and their families knowing I had a serious, lifelong illness mortified me. I didn't want to be the sick kid. I didn't want to be the diseased dude. I just wanted to be the normal guitar-playing, skateboarding teen I felt I deserved to be.

Like most teenagers, I wanted to be both perfectly normal *and* totally unique at the same time. I wanted to both fit in *and* separate myself from the pack. Admitting to myself that I had Behcet's disease meant fitting in and being normal were no longer on the table. The diagnosis made me feel abnormal and different from my peers. So instead of accepting the cold, hard truth, I just pretended like it didn't exist. My philosophy was simple: deny till you die about the knee, the sores, and the eye.

We all lie to ourselves. We all refuse to believe certain things because they're too embarrassing or painful. Sometimes they're little things, sometimes big. Sometimes we get over them and eventually find acceptance, sometimes we don't. Sometimes we even carry that denial with us all the way to the grave. It took me a long time to accept that I had Behcet's disease. I was in denial for years. But when I finally accepted it, I felt like a huge weight had been lifted off my shoulders.

There's some value to the saying, "The truth will set you free." I don't think Jesus was talking about being honest with yourself about having Behcet's disease when he said it in John 8:32, but it's certainly true in this case. When I did finally start to accept the truth, it was incredibly liberating. That acceptance would unlock a whole new world of of experiences, knowledge, and opportunities. And it would finally put an end to the unrelenting anxiety of always trying to keep my illness hidden. It takes a lot of effort to hide something from yourself when you know deep down it's true.

Unfortunately, fully accepting that I had Behcet's disease was still years away. What *wasn't* years away: more symptoms, more suffering, and a lot more denial.

"My doctor is nice; every time I see him, I'm ashamed of what I think of doctors in general." - Mignon McLaughlin

8. Sacked

After Dr. Woods diagnosed me with Behcet's disease, he referred me to a rheumatologist. These are specialists who treat autoimmune and musculoskeletal conditions, which have traditionally been known as rheumatic diseases. The last thing I wanted in my life was another doctor I'd have to regularly see. But I agreed and soon started seeing a rheumatologist – or rheumy for short.

I couldn't help myself from letting at least a little chuckle slip out whenever I heard his name. Not only would my new rheumy's name be funny to just about any sixteen-year-old young man, it was especially funny to me. It almost felt like the universe was making a big low-brow joke at my expense. My new rheumatologist was named after one of the most-painful symptoms I had – or at least the body part it affected.

His name was Dr. Sack.

I found it absolutely hilarious that the doctor I had to see for the sores on my nutsack had Sack for a last name. The first year I saw him, I couldn't say it with a straight face. I can't imagine it could've been easy going through life, especially high school, with a last name like that.

Dr. Burton Sack was a well-known and well-respected rheumatologist, known and respected by his peers and patients alike. Eventually, I'd become one of those patients who liked and respected him. It would've been hard not to. Dr. Sack was a highly competent and compassionate physician. Friendly guy, too. Very easy to get along with. His pleasant personality made it much easier for my insecure teenage self to whip out my balls so he could see how severe the ulcers were. Dr. Sack was in his late fifties when I first started seeing him in 1997. He had a full head of white hair always entered the exam room with a smile.

When I first met Dr. Sack, I was a fucking mess. I limped into his office on crutches, still recovering from knee surgery. My left pupil was more than twice the size of my right from the eye drops Dr. Woods had prescribed. The vision in my left eye was still blurry. I had a mouthful of oral ulcers. I had a crotchful of genital ulcers. And there was one more symptom – perhaps the worst of all – that I brought with me everywhere I went: my lousy attitude.

I was in constant pain. My mouth hurt. My nuts hurt. My knee still hurt. My joints hurt. When everything hurts, it's hard to be a big ball of sunshine. I was miserable and it showed. Dr. Sack, being the caring and compassionate man he was, could see my suffering from a mile away. He prescribed me several medications to try to control my illness. Off the top of my head, within the first year of seeing him I remember being put on (more) prednisone, methotrexate, colchicine, folic acid, dapsone, and tetracycline. He also prescribed something for all the pain: extra-strength Vicodin (Vicodin ES)[1] – and lots of them.

---

[1] Vicodin ES contains two ingredients: the opioid hydrocodone (7.5 mg) and acetaminophen (750 mg), the active ingredient in Tylenol. Regular-strength Vicodin contains 5 mg of hydrocodone and 500 mg of acetaminophen.

Back in the eighties and nineties, Vicodin was considered to be a much-safer, less-addictive alternative to other opioids like morphine and codeine. Unsurprisingly, drug companies were responsible – at least in part – for spreading the idea. Now we now know this to be absolute horseshit. Hydrocodone, the main ingredient in Vicodin, is just as addictive as any other opioid. But back then it was considered to be more-or-less risk free and Dr. Sack used to prescribe them to my by the hundreds.

In 2014, the Drug Enforcement Administration (DEA) switched Vicodin from being a Schedule III substance to Schedule II, a much-stricter designation. Schedule III substances can be prescribed with refills while Schedule II substances require a new prescription every month. Back in the 1990s and early 2000s when I was on them, I'd get prescriptions for 150 Vicodin ES, each with six refills. That's a lot of extra-strength Vikes.

At first it was great. Just one-half of a pill made my mouth and balls feel better for hours. It put me in a better mood and made me less anxious. I could eat, be social with friends, and even brush my teeth without wanting to scream at the top of my lungs. After being in more-or-less constant pain for years, it was nice.

For a long time after going on Vicodin ES, I actually took less than I'd been prescribed. The bottle said to take one-to-two tablets every four-to-six hours. But I only took half a tab every four-or-five hours. It was enough to give me the pain relief I so desperately craved. Over time, I'd gradually need more and more to get the same analgesic effect. That's just the way opioids work. But for the better part of a year, a half-tab of Vicodin ES was all I needed to feel halfway decent.

It was in June of 1997 that I got hit with the inflammation in my right knee and left eye. I ended up just barely finishing my junior year of high school. I'd missed a lot of days during the school year, especially in that last month before summer break. I suspect that I only passed because some of my teachers felt bad for me and gave me a higher grade than I'd earned. Of course I was happy to pass. But I hated the idea of getting special treatment because people felt bad for me. It wasn't the special treatment part I had a problem with. That's all good. It was the feeling bad part that I hated. I didn't want anyone to feel bad for me as a teenager and I don't want anyone to feel bad for me now.

By the time the summer came to an end and it was time to start my senior year of high school, my right knee was back to normal. The crutches were long gone and so were the achy armpits that went along with them. I still got oral and genital ulcers, but the Vicodin usually took the edge off. And my left eye was doing a lot better. I no longer had to use the eye drops. So no more big pupil, small pupil. The vision in my left eye hadn't totally returned to normal and it never would. But by September of 1997, it was nowhere near as blurry as it had been in June. Dr. Woods, in an August follow-up appointment, told me he was surprised by how well it'd recovered. He thought that since I'd refused the eye injection he recommended, it wouldn't heal nearly as well as it did. As you might imagine, I was quite happy to prove him wrong.

Getting through the first-three years of public high school was not easy. By the time I made it to my senior year, I'd had enough. I'm sure high school would've sucked even if I'd been perfectly healthy. But being forced to go with Behcet's disease, as I had been for the previous three years, was torturous. Every single day was an overwhelming struggle and I'd had enough. So I stopped going.

    I think I made it through a total of one-half-of-one day of my senior year. For the first couple weeks of school, I'd get up, get ready, get picked up by a friend, and then we'd just drive around listening to music, drinking coffee, and smoking cigarettes for a few hours. Then when we were sure our parents had left for work, he'd drop me off at home and head to his own. Of course, it wasn't long before the school contacted both of our parents. But those were a couple of great weeks. He'd drop me off and I'd have the whole house to myself until the late afternoon. That gave me plenty of time to; play my guitar at full volume; smoke cigarettes out on the front porch; find, use, and carefully put back one of my dad's porno mags; find, eat, and carefully put back some of the snacks my mother kept hidden; and take a nice long nap before anyone came home.

    I was still several months away from being an adult, but you only have to be sixteen to drop out of school in Massachusetts. So that's what I did. My parents were furious. But they got mad at me so often that, by then, it didn't really phase me. They told me that I needed to go to school if I wanted to keep living there. So I found the perfect solution: night school.

    Night school was fucking awesome. Three hours a night, two nights a week – that's it. I got to sleep in every morning and wake up feeling rested. Having to get up at 6AM for the first three years of high school made me feel even worse than I already did. Being able to sleep in made a huge difference to my mood and energy levels. The students who went to night school were an interesting mix of burnouts, misfits, delinquents, and others who couldn't hack it in normal high school. There were even a few people who went there because of health problems like me. A young woman who had Lupus comes to mind, but there were others. I had several friends who went to night school, including my good friend Malinda. I used to picked her up on my way in and drop her off afterward. Night school was better than regular school in every possible way. They even let us smoke outside between classes.

And then there were the girls.

There were plenty of cute girls in my regular high school, but nothing like night school. Those girls were on a whole other level. There were a few in particular who were drop-dead gorgeous, the hottest women I'd ever seen in my entire life up to that point. I didn't have the balls to actually *talk* to them, but I was just happy to be able to *look* at them. Suzanne, the hottest of the hot, talked to *me* one time and I'll never forget it.

"You walk slow," she said from behind me as I worked my way up the stairs to the second-floor sociology class we had together.

"I'm sorry," I replied, looking back but not making eye contact with her or her friend.

Both Suzanne and her almost-but-not-quite-as-hot friend laughed. My knees got weak and I wanted to curl up in the corner of the stairwell and magically disappear, I was so embarrassed.

"You don't have to be sorry," Suzanne said, still laughing a little bit.

That was the extent of our conversation. I don't remember a single thing that I learned in any of my night-school classes, but I remember every word of that short conversation with Suzanne. I shouldn't have apologized for walking slowly, but it just slipped out. Maybe I should've said something like, "You'd be walking slowly, too, if you had a quarter-sized ulcer on your balls rubbing against your leg with each step." Had I actually said that, perhaps she'd still remember *me* all these years later.

Dropping out of high school and going to night school was one of the best decisions I've ever made. The best part of all? I graduated six-months earlier than I would've had I stayed at my public high school. And I didn't get a GED or some other equivalency certificate. I got an actual high school diploma. Night school was less days a week, less hours a day, and less months a year but resulted in the same diploma. My only regret was that I didn't discover night school sooner like Malinda had.

I didn't have a graduation party. I did, however, get a fun graduation present from my body a couple months later – a present that would land me in the hospital for the better part of a week.

> "In the midst of winter, I found there was, within me, an infinite summer." - Albert Camus

9. Clot

Some people, when diagnosed with a chronic illness like Behcet's, let it control their lives. They hand over the reigns to the disease and say, "Here you go. It's all yours!" They cater to its every whim; every flare[1]; every ache and pain; every symptom, no matter how minor. They use their diagnosis as an excuse to stay out of the action, watching life pass them by from the safety of the sidelines. They avoid chasing even their most coveted desires, letting their dreams slowly fade into oblivion. They play the perpetual victim role, surrendering all hope and all power to their diagnosis.

I'm not one of those people.

Now let me be perfectly clear: I'm not judging anyone. I get it. I do. Having this disease – or any chronic illness – fucking sucks. I wouldn't wish it upon my worst enemy. There have been times when I've felt defeated, depressed, helpless, and hopeless. During my teens, on more than one occasion I remember actually raising my fist to the sky and cursing any god who would inflict such suffering on one of his children. I completely understand why so many people give up, give in, and surrender to this shitty disease and others like it.

But I refuse to be one of them.

When I was still a teenager, I made the conscious decision to never, ever – not even for a

---

[1] A "flare" or "flare up" is a common way of saying that symptoms of a disease are either appearing or worsening.

second – let this disease dictate how I live my life. I refused to let it run my life then and I refuse to let it run my life now. Instead of living on the disease's terms, I would live my life the way I wanted to in spite of this dreadful illness. But it hasn't always been easy.

About two months after graduating from night school, I was finishing up a shift at McDonald's. I'd been working there for over a year at that point. As soon as my shift was over, I went out back to the employee break room to get changed. There was a party going on down the street I couldn't wait to get to and the last thing I wanted to do was show up in my McDonald's uniform. Getting undressed was easy enough. I pulled my green, grease-splotched shirt over my head and put it on the table. Then without bending over – not that I could've if I'd wanted to – I kicked off my sneakers, undid my belt, and let my black Dickies fall to the floor. That was the easy part. I knew getting dressed would prove to be more of a challenge. I tried to change quickly so no one would see me, but it wasn't quick enough. A buddy of mine who got off at the same time walked into the break room to grab his stuff.

"What the fuck is wrong with your leg?" Jimi asked the second he walking into the break room.

"Nothing. I'm fine," I replied.

"Bro, your left leg is twice the size of your right one."

"It's nothing, really."

"Whatever, dude," Jimi said, shaking his head. "You going to Daren's party?"

"You know it! After as I get dressed and punch out, I'm gonna walk over there. I should be at Daren's apartment in about ten, fifteen minutes tops.

You're going, I take it?"

"Yeah, I'll be there," Jimi replied, taking his Cooler Than Smack[2] cassette out of the break room boombox that'd been blasting all night. "I gotta run home real quick and then I'll be over in like a half."

"Cool," I said, refolding my McDonald's shirt for the third time, trying to stall until Jimi left the break room. I didn't want him to see me getting dressed. "See you there."

"You sure you're all good?" Jimi asked, his eyes fixed on my swollen leg.

"Yeah," I answered, then quickly changed the subject. "I bet Daren's party is gonna be off the chain. I know Trista, Pepin, Daren's brother, and all three Heathers are gonna be there."

"Oh shit! Heather Samba is going?" Jimi asked, his face lighting up like the two-hundred-foot-tall McDonald's sign out in front of the restaurant. "Maybe I should take a quick shower while I'm home. Alright bro, see you in a bit."

"Later."

Once Jimi was out of the break room, I pulled my jeans out of the backpack that always went everywhere with me. To this day, I still never leave home without my trusty backpack. You never know when you're going to need to re-deodorize, brush your teeth, put on a fresh pair of socks, or down half a bottle of Pepto-Bismol when out of nowhere and for no apparent reason the Behcet's decides to make your stomach feel like you ate a lit firecracker. Pulling the jeans out of the backpack was the easy part. Getting

---

[2] Cooler Than Smack was a local rap group from Brockton, MA. The cassette was The Disco Dust Delight, a six-song EP. I still have a copy of it from more than twenty-years ago. Good shit.

them on my body would prove to be much more of a challenge.

Jimi wasn't kidding. My left leg was almost twice the size of my right. Little did I know that I had massive blood clots going all the way down my leg. I could barely move the thing. It was as stiff as a board and felt like like it weighed five-hundred pounds. I'm sure a normal seventeen-year-old would've probably gone to the hospital when it first started swelling up a few days earlier. But I'd been having weird stuff like that happen to me for as long as I could remember. One time my thumb swelled up to twice its normal size for no apparent reason over the course of about a day only to return to normal a day later. On several occasions my arm would get really, *really* stiff, worsening over the course of a few days. Then over the course of a few more, it would gradually return to normal. Shit like that happened to me all the time. I figured if I just ignored my swollen leg long enough, if I gave it enough time, eventually it would return to normal on its own.

I figured wrong.

With my jeans in hand, I tried to bend over to put them on. I only made it about halfway down. Normal means of getting dressed weren't going to work so I had to get creative. I dropped my jeans on the break-room floor and stepped my left foot into the left leg, wiggling my foot until the jeans were around my ankle. Then I sat down in one of the break-room chairs and threw my left leg up on the table – literally threw it. My leg felt so heavy that I needed to use both hands to launch it up onto the table. I reached up and tried to grab my jeans, but they were just out of reach. More wiggling was in order. Using my hands once again, I used them to jiggle my jeans up my leg until I could reach them. Once I could, I slipped my right foot into the other leg and finally pulled them all the way up. Then I pushed my leg off the table, letting it slam to the floor.

Almost there. All I needed to do was get my sneakers on and I could be on my way to the party. I got the right one on no problem. The left was more of a challenge. I was able to get the sneaker on my foot by standing up, sticking my toes in it, and doing some more wiggling until my whole foot was in. But it quickly became clear that tying it was beyond my capability.

"Hey!" I yelled as a coworker walked past the break room.

"Were you talking to me?" Krista asked, taking a few steps backward, poking her head through the break-room door.

"I was, yes," I replied. "Do me a quick favor?"

"What?"

"Tie my sneaker for me?"

Krista didn't reply. She just eyed me up and down suspiciously.

"Please?" I begged.

"Why can't you do it?" she asked, still giving me a look.

"I twisted my knee skateboarding and I can't bend it."

"Okay," Krista replied and smiled. She looked up at me while tying my sneaker and said, "You always seem to be getting busted up skating."

"That's what happens when you're trying to learn new tricks. It's part of the fun. Thanks."

"No problem," she replied, getting up and disappearing out the break room door.

Skateboarding remained my go-to explanation for many of my strange Behcet's-related symptoms. Everyone knew I liked to skateboard, so no one questioned it. It had been almost nine months since my last "skateboarding injury," the inflammation in my right knee.

Now fully dressed, I grabbed my backpack and worked my way through the maze of the grill area and up to the front of the restaurant. Making sure it was the absolute last thing I did before leaving, I punched out at one of the unattended registers. I still remember my employee number: 667. I'd tried to get Diana, the manager, to change it to 666, a number universally admired by rebellious teens everywhere. But she explained to me that employee numbers were randomly assigned and couldn't be changed. 667 wasn't nearly as cool, but at least it was easy to remember.

I left McDonald's and started walking to Daren's apartment. It was a walk I'd made many times before. He lived in the same apartment complex that my ex-girlfriend Heather did. She'd also be at the party. If I really took my sweet-ass time, at most the walk should've taken me fifteen minutes. But on that bone-chilling February night, it took a lot longer. I made the first quarter of the journey without much trouble. But then my left leg started getting *really* heavy. It had been feeling heavy for days, but not like this. The stiffness and soreness was no longer just in my leg. My lower back was also killing me. Every step got harder and harder until the pain was so unbearable that I couldn't walk at all.

I did the only thing I really could do: sit down. If I'd had a cell phone, I could've called someone to come pick me up. But it was 1998 and the only electronics I had on me were my pager and my Walkman, neither of which would've been much help. So I just sat on the side of the road in the the freezing cold.

    I remember feeling really anxious as I sat there shivering. It probably should've been my stiff leg, sore back, or the very real threat of hypothermia that I was worrying about. But none of those things weighed very heavily on my mind. I was worried I wouldn't get to Darren's party in time to put in my order with whoever was going to the packie.[1]

    After sitting for a few minutes, my leg and back started to feel a little better. I got up and continued down the sidewalk. Like before, after putting another quarter of the distance to Darren's behind me, the unbearable pain returned. I had no choice but to stop and sit down again. My nose, ears, and fingers were so cold they felt like if you hit them hard enough they would've shattered. But that was nothing compared to the pain in my lower back. As I'd eventually find out, it wasn't just my leg that had blood clots in it. My inferior vena cava, the large vein that carries blood from the lower half of my body directly to my heart, also had a massive clot in it.

    A few minutes later, I got up and continued on my way. This time, I was only able to travel about one-eighth of the distance before I had to sit down again. After a few minutes of sitting, I got up and and kept going. And after a couple minutes of walking, I had to sit down again. The process of walking until the pain was unbearable, sitting down for a few minutes, then getting up and continuing on my way

---

[1]   Packie is Massachusetts talk for package store, otherwise known as a liquor store.

until the pain got bad again went on until I got to Daren's apartment. What should've taken me no more than fifteen minutes ended up taking almost forty-five.

    I limped my way up the stairs to Daren's second-floor apartment. With only a few minutes left until the packie closed, I was sure I'd missed my chance to put in an order. When I hobbled into Daren's apartment, once I got through the huge cloud of cigarette-and-pot smoke, I was very happy to see that his older brother was getting ready to make the last booze run of the night. I'd had more than enough time to think about what I wanted during my extended walk, so I scribbled it all down and handed him the paper and some money as he was on his way out the door. Then I flopped down on the couch, relieved knowing I wouldn't have to walk anywhere else for the rest of the night.

    I was determined to get to Daren's party no matter what. A few blood clots in my leg and under my heart weren't going to stop me. They certain didn't make getting there any easier. But I didn't let them stop me. I did what I wanted to do in spite of the disease that I'd been diagnosed with just nine-months earlier. I refused to let it control me then and I refuse to let it control me now.

    Daren's party was a fucking blast. I had a great time with a lot of friends, made out with a cute girl I'd never met before, drank until I blacked out (and then drank some more), and then spent some quality time in the bathroom hugging the bowl until I eventually passed out. It was a good night, a night like many others I'd had before and would have again.

    Something interesting happened once I started drinking and I wouldn't fully understand why until years later. The more I drank, the better my back and leg felt. Not only did they feel better, the swelling went down considerably. At the time, I just assumed they felt better because that's what alcohol does – it makes you feel better. But the alcohol didn't just make my leg and back *feel* better. It *actually* made them better.

The girl I'd been making out with at the party and I left Daren's apartment for a while and went for a walk. By that point I was totally shitfaced. The whole time we were out, my leg and back felt fine. They didn't start swelling up like they had when I walked from McDonald's to Daren's. At the time, I didn't think much of it. But now I understand what was going on.

Blood clots clog up your vessels, restricting blood flow. That's why they put you on blood thinners when you're diagnosed with them. While blood thinners don't actually thin your blood – not exactly – they do allow your blow to flow easier without clotting up. You know what else does that? Alcohol. It does it well and it does it fast. I drank so much at Daren's party, my blood would've been flowing like a waterfall.

On the surface, I was just a teen trying to get fucked up and have a good time. But unknowingly, I was using a common-but-powerful drug, ethanol, to temporarily treat my symptoms. The next morning when I woke up, my leg and back still felt fine. Even after having puked several times, I'd drank so much the night before that there was still plenty of alcohol floating around in my system. But over the course of the day, the swelling and pain slowly returned.

I don't remember if it was the day after Daren's party or the day after that, but eventually the pain and swelling got so bad that I did the last thing I wanted to do: I told my parents. They immediately brought me to Morton Hospital where I'd end up spending the better part of a week. Though I don't recall if it was that Saturday or Sunday I told my folks, it was definitely on the weekend. So they couldn't just bring me to my pediatrician and had to take me to the emergency room.

    In retrospect, I should've gone to the hospital or at least to see my doctor long before I *actually* ended up going. I should've called in sick to work and I should've skipped Daren's party. It wasn't his first party and I knew it wouldn't be the last. Parties at Daren's happened all the time. But I was determined to go and no amount of pain and embarrassment was going to stop me.

    Now that I'm older, I'm much better at thinking long term. If I was to find myself in the same situation now that I did that night, I'd skip the party, skip work, and go straight to the hospital. I would know there'd be other parties and that McDonald's wasn't going anywhere. But at the time, those things were important to me and I was determined to not let my illness stop me from doing them. Though I'm much older and wiser with different priorities now, my attitude hasn't changed. I still refuse to let my diagnosis prevent me from doing the things in life that I want to do.

    But I've learned to take it one step further. Not only do I refuse to let Behcet's prevent me from doing what I want to do, I use it to motivate me to actually do those things. This disease has lit a fire under my ass that pushes me to live each day to the fullest because it could be the last day I can.

    I was about six months from my eighteenth

birthday when I got the clots. I'd already become sexually active, losing my virginity almost a year earlier.

  Sex? Check.

  My Vicodin popping continued. I loved getting drunk with friends. And rarely but occasionally I'd smoke some weed.

  Drugs? Check.

  The only thing missing from my life was a little rock and roll.

"I want to rock and roll all night and party every day." - Kiss

10. Rock & Roll

While still going to night school, I joined a band. This one wasn't a marching band – it was a rock band. If I'm ever asked to join another marching band, I'm marching in the opposite direction double time. And in this band I didn't play drums – I played lead guitar.

As a kid, my parents made me take piano lessons. Sometimes I loved them, sometimes I hated them – but I'll always be thankful for them. Those lessons gave me a solid musical foundation to build upon. After a few years of piano lessons, I took a couple years of drum lessons. Then at the age of thirteen, I borrowed a cheap, beat-up acoustic guitar from a friend and taught myself how to play. Between the piano and drum lessons, I was able to pick up the guitar pretty quickly.

I loved being in a band – a *real* band. This wasn't just a high school band or a go-nowhere garage band that only played in front of friends and family. I mean, I guess we were a basement band when I first joined, technically. But it wouldn't be long before we'd start renting a room at a nearby rehearsal studio called River's Edge. Dozens of bands, some of them nationally-touring acts, practiced there. For a live-music lover like myself, River's Edge was a great place to be. I loved watching the other bands practice. And it wouldn't be long after getting our room at the studio that my band began playing gigs around New England.

None of the guys knew that I had Behcet's.

There were five of us in the band, one of which I became very close with. But I never told any of them. I didn't want to come across as weak. I didn't want to be *the sick one*. I guess I thought it would be better to be *the one who always had lame excuses for his strange behavior*. I was like Sabrina the Teenage Witch always having to explain the strange things happening around her. The only difference, I wasn't trying to hide the fact that I could use magic – I was trying to hide the fact that I had a chronic illness. And I didn't have to explain the strange things happening *around* me. I had to explain the strange things happening *to* me.

"Where have you been?" Herbie, the band's drummer and member I was closest with, asked over the phone. "I've been trying to get ahold of you for days. We all have. You missed practice the other night."

"I know," I replied, my voice a little shaky. "I'm sorry I missed practice. I'm actually in the hospital right now. That's why I wasn't there. I've been here since Sunday."

"Oh my god," Herbie said with genuine concern. "Are you alright? Why are you in the hospital?"

"I fucked myself up skateboarding," I lied. "But I'll be fine. I should be out in a day or two."

"Do you want me to come visit you? Do you want me to get the guys together so we can all come see you?"

"No!" I shouted. A nurse poked her head into the room to make sure I was alright. Calmer, I continued, "No, that's not necessary. Like I said, I'll be out soon. But I won't be at practice tonight."

"Obviously. Is there anything I can do for

you?" Herbie asked. He was a good friend, a good bandmate, and a good dude in general. I could tell he really cared.

"No, thank you. I've got everything I need," I replied, looking down at my Sony Walkman and the small stack of punk rock cassettes my mother had brought me from home. "I'll call you when I'm out of this shithole."

"Okay, cool. Feel better."

"Thanks, man. Tell the guys I said hi and I'll be at practice next week. Peace."

"Later."

I hadn't used the skateboarding excuse on Herbie and the other guys in the band before. It worked like a charm. None of them suspected I had multiple blood clots in one of my legs and in my inferior vena cava caused by the lifelong autoimmune disease I'd been diagnosed with a year earlier. They thought I simply injured myself skating.

A day or two after Daren's party, I showed my swollen leg to my parents and they took me to Morton Hospital. The doctors immediately suspected one or more blood clots, started me on a heparin[1] drip, and gave me Percocet for the pain. But when they wheeled me down to the radiology department in the basement for an ultrasound, it came back negative. I've had several ultrasounds over the years, but none quite like that first one.

Think about baseball, I thought to myself as the attractive, young sonographer slowly dragged the ultrasound probe up my leg toward my crotch. *Think about skateboarding. Think about something –*

---

[1] Heparin is an anticoagulant (blood thinner) used to treat and prevent blood clots.

anything – non-sexual. Just don't get hard. Do. Not. Get. Hard.

"It feels strange, I know," the woman said in response to what I have to imagine was a bizarre look on my face – the look of a horny teenager doing everything he could to stay flaccid while a hot, older woman was touching him. "But you're doing great, sweetie."

I repeat: Do not get hard! I thought as her hand moved farther north up my leg. *Just because she called me "sweetie" doesn't mean she likes me. Just because she's getting close to my dick doesn't mean she wants to see it grow to its full glory. She's just doing her job. No need to get aroused. Please oh please do not get hard!*

"Thank you," I replied.

The sonographer ran the probe up my leg over the slimy jelly she'd smeared all over it. When she got to my upper, inner thigh, it sent a tingle right to my you-know-what. The only thing I had on was a pair of boxer shorts that had been pulled to the side so the sonographer had access to my entire leg. They were covering my junk, but just barely. One of my balls must've been peeking out because when she ran the probe from my leg up to my abdomen, I felt her hand gently brush the side of it.

Don't get hard. Don't get hard. Don't get hard, I repeated in my head over and over.

It took every ounce of self control in my entire being, but I did it: I made it through the ultrasound without getting an erection. When the attractive sonographer's hand brushed against me, I must've flinched or made a face. I looked up at her immediately after and she cracked what was almost a half-smile, but not quite. Maybe a one-third smile. A full smile would've been too obvious. Even a half-smile would've been too suggestive. The corners of her mouth just barely jumped up for a second, letting *me* know that *she* knew the brief ball brush had an effect on me. Maybe she did it on purpose. Maybe she was *trying* to turn me on. Or maybe I was just a horny teenager still inexperienced enough that everything down there was super sensitive to any kind of touch.

    I have to admit, for a medical procedure, the ultrasound felt really good. The jelly rubbed all over me by a hot older woman, the dim lighting of the exam room, the feeling of skin-on-skin as her knuckles brushed my testicles: all of it drove me wild. Whether the sonographer was trying to turn me on or not, she definitely did. But I somehow managed to control myself – until I got wheeled back up to my room. As soon as I was alone, I got as hard as a rock. Taking my IV cart with me, I limped into the bathroom and let all the fantasies I'd fought off during the ultrasound run freely through my mind. Maybe two minutes later – if that – I came out of the bathroom, laid down, shut my eyes, and slept ultra-soundly all night.

    When the ultrasound came back negative, the doctors were at a loss as to what to do with me. It was obvious that *something* was wrong. All signs pointed to one-or-more blood clots but none of the tests revealed any. My leg and back were feeling better with every passing day being on heparin. I wanted to get out of the hospital so I could get back to playing guitar, smoking weed, and chasing girls. But one of the doctors at the hospital insisted I stay and get one more test: an MRI.

    That doctor is now my rheumatologist, a man I both like and respect. But at the time I resented the shit out of him. How dare he keep me in the hospital for an extra day or two? The other doctors were fine with sending me home. Why did he have to convince my parents to keep me there longer?

Because he cared, that's why. Because he knew I had blood clots somewhere and was determined to find them. There are two qualities I have come to look for in a physician: competence and compassion. Most doctors have one or the other. Some have neither. Dr. Kieval is that rare breed of doctor who has both. I didn't appreciate him for it when we first met but I'd come to eventually.

The MRI revealed what none of the other tests did: that I had multiple clots in my left leg and in my inferior vena cava. You'd think that the MRI results would've changed the way I felt about Dr. Kieval keeping me in the hospital longer, but I resented him for years after that. To be fair, though, I also resented both of my parents, many of my teachers, and plenty of other people, too. I was a resentful teen. When you're in pain all the time, it's easy to be bitter.

After spending the better part of a week in the hospital, they finally discharged me. I still remember having that first cigarette as soon as I got home. Several doctors made it clear to me that I shouldn't smoke with blood clots. And I made it perfectly clear to them that I wasn't going to listen. After not having a cigarette for almost a week, it was incredibly satisfying, if not a little disgusting. Within a couple of days, I was right back to smoking a pack a day.

Over the next several weeks, my leg and back continued to get better. After a couple of months, my leg was almost back to its normal size – but not quite. For the next eighteen years, my left leg would be slightly larger than my right. Few people ever noticed, but I was always very aware of the difference. Fortunately, they're now back to being the same size. Eighteen years after the clots in my left leg, I got clots in my right, which balanced them out.

I continued to play guitar in that band for about six more months until they kicked me out. Herbie tried to convince the others to let me stay but they insisted I leave. Why? Because I'm an asshole. I'd been running my mouth about how I thought the singer was a fat piece of shit who couldn't sing. Being fat had nothing to do with my growing dislike of him, but I threw it in there anyway. *Fat piece of shit* had a little extra zing to it compared to just *piece of shit*. It did in 1998, anyway. Nowadays, you can't call someone a fat piece of shit without catching quite a bit of shit yourself. In my defense, he did go by the name Fat Mike. He called himself fat plenty of times before I ever did. Regardless, I was a dick and they had every right to throw me out of the band.

If I'm being honest, it stung a little bit. I felt like a jerk because I'd been acting like one. A few years later, I apologized to Fat Mike and the other guys. We're all on good terms now and keep in touch on Facebook. That band broke up just a few months after kicking me out. Though I couldn't have known it at the time, they actually did me a huge favor. Had they not kicked me out when they did, I would've missed out on a big opportunity that was right around the corner.

"Here I am on the road again. There I am up on the stage. Here I go playing the star again. There I go. Turn the page." - Bob Seger

11. Drained

More than half a year had gone by since I was hospitalized with the clots. During that time I didn't experience any new Behcet's symptoms. Just the occasional genital-or-oral ulcer. I continued to hang out at the studio where my now-former band practiced. I had friends in several other bands and liked to watch them practice. One of those bands, a nationally touring act that had just been signed to a New York record label, lost their bass player not long after I was booted out of my first band. They'd just recorded an album for their new label and were getting ready to go on a two-week East Coast tour to promote it. Though I was mainly known throughout the studio as a lead guitarist, it was also known that I could play bass, drums, and piano. They asked me if I wanted to audition and I jumped on the opportunity. I'd been a fan of theirs for years. I learned a bunch of their songs, tried out, they liked me, and asked me to join the next day. Of course, I said yes.

A couple weeks later, I was thousands of miles from home on tour with my new band. I'd just turned eighteen a few months earlier and was the youngest member. I was by far the heaviest drinker in the band which was ironic since I was the only member who wasn't over twenty-one. Had I not been in the band, most of the clubs we played at wouldn't have even let me in. But since I *was* with the band, not only did I get in, most places gave me a bracelet that let me drink for free. Open bar night after night.

It was great – at first.

Being on the road is hard. It's a lot of fun, but it's hard. You're away from your friends and family, you're stuck in a van with the same five sweaty dudes twenty-four hours a day, your diet consists of fast food and truck stop snacks, and you never stay in one place long enough to truly relax. When you throw free alcohol into the mix, it's a recipe for disaster. The booze makes you miss your friends and family even more, it makes you fight with your fellow bandmates and, of course, it's no better for your body than Burger King, Taco Bell, or truck stop food.

I refilled my Vicodin ES and other meds the day before leaving to go on that first tour. Throughout the whole thing, I was popping Vicodin all day and getting drunk every night. I did my best to be discreet about the pill popping, but sometimes it wasn't possible. When you're in the back row of the van wedged between the singer and a roadie for four hours at a time, it's hard to do much of anything without someone noticing.

"What was that?" the singer asked.

"What was what?" I replied, as if I didn't know exactly what he was talking about.

"Those pills. I just saw you pop three pills. What were they?"

"Oh, those? Just ibuprofen."

"What do you need ibuprofen for?" the singer asked.

"What are you, my doctor?" I shot back.

"I'm just wondering, man. You don't have to be a dick about it. Excuse me for being concerned."

"You're not concerned. No matter what answer I give you, you're going to give me shit about it cause that's what you do."

You see, the singer was straightedge. That means he abstained from all drugs and alcohol. If that's how you want to live your life, cool. I have no problem with anyone being straightedge in principle. But a lot of straightedge people I've met feel the constant need to judge those of us who like to pop the occasional pill (or three) and have the occasional drink (or ten). And the singer used to judge me all the time for drinking, smoking cigarettes, and popping what he thought were ibuprofen. It drove me crazy. He wasn't the only one throwing judgments around, though. I used to judge him, too. He had a wonderful girlfriend back home, yet cheated on her every night when we were on the road. I hated that about him. If he hadn't given *me* such a hard time, I probably wouldn't have cared about what *he* was doing. But I needed something to judge him about for judging me and I chose that. Don't judge.

Being on the road is tough enough as it is. But being on the road with someone you don't get along with sucks. After we got back from that first tour, I didn't see or talk to any of my bandmates for a week. We always took a week off from practicing when we got back from a tour. After spending all day everyday with the same guys for weeks at a time, they're the last people you want to spend time with when you get home. I spent much of that week going back and forth between my bedroom and bathroom. As soon as we got back, my Vicodin prescription ran out and I couldn't refill it yet. This was the beginning of a vicious cycle I'd continue for years.

The pharmacy would let me refill my Vicodin prescription every twenty-three days. Like clockwork, I'd be there on the twenty-third day as soon as they opened. I'd get my hundred-and-fifty Vicodin ES and walk out the door with a big, goofy smile on my face, knowing that I'd be feeling good for the next several days. The prescription would run out before I could refill it and I'd go into opioid withdrawal. For the next few days I'd have cold sweats, diarrhea, and be incredibly depressed. Then just as I was starting to feel normal, I'd refill my prescription and start the cycle all over again. Every cycle, I'd tear through my prescription just a little faster than the one before. By the time I was in my twenties, all hundred-and-fifty extra-strength Vicodin would be gone in less than a week.

After we took a week off to recover from that first East Coast tour, the band resumed our normal three-day-a-week practice schedule. But when we returned, there were only four of us, not five.

"Where's Neil?" I asked. Not only was he missing, his guitar and Marshall half-stack[1] wasn't there, either.

"He quit," the drummer answered.

"What? Why?"

"Cause he's a little bitch," the singer replied.

"He wants to settle down with his girlfriend and can't do that being on the road all the time," the drummer said.

"Oh. That sucks," I replied, doing my best to hide how happy the news made me. It wasn't that I didn't like Neil. He and I got along just fine. But I would've rather been playing guitar in the band than bass and I was happy to hear that we apparently had a vacancy. "So who's going to take Neil's place?"

"We haven't had a chance to even talk about it

---

[1] A guitar amplifier. Marshall's among the top brands. Great sounding amps. I had one myself at the time.

yet," the drummer answered. "He just told me that he was quitting yesterday."

"Let me guess," the remaining guitar player said. "You want the position?"

"Yes," I replied, still trying to hide my enthusiasm.

"I'm okay with you switching to guitar," the drummer and de facto leader of the band said. "But there's a problem. Then we need to find a new bass player. And it's a hell of a lot easier to find a guitarist than a bassist."

"If I find us a new bass player," I suggested, "can I come on as the second guitarist?"

The drummer looked first to the singer, then to the guitar player, and finally to me.

"Sure," he said after getting two nods.

"Cool," I replied, unable to stop the corners of my mouth from jumping up.

Before practice was over, I had a list of prospective bass players in my head. As soon as we were done, I scoured the studio for any bandless bassists I could find. It took some convincing and a six pack of Sam Adams, but I managed to convince my buddy Justin to join the band. It was a win-win situation. Not only did it allow me to switch to guitar, having Justin on the road with us gave me someone to drink with. Starting with our next practice session a couple days later, I was officially the band's second lead guitarist.

Justin was a social drinker. He'd buy a six pack before practice and only drink two or three of them. Since I was still only eighteen, I couldn't buy alcohol myself. But Justin and several others down at the studio were cool enough to buy booze for me. I remember always thinking, *When I'm over twenty-*

one, I'll buy alcohol for anyone who asks to make up for all the people who bought for me when I was underage. Well, aside from a few isolated times when I bought for underage friends in my early twenties, I've never purchased alcohol for anyone under twenty-one. Buying alcohol for someone that is not of age is a serious offense here in Massachusetts. If I was going to get in trouble for something booze related, you'd better believe I'd be the one drinking it.

    Having Justin on the road with me made touring much more fun. The singer and drummer didn't drink or smoke and the other guitarist only smoked weed. But Justin and I both drank and smoked cigarettes. It was great not being the only one holding up the van because they were finishing off a butt. And the singer gave me much less shit with Justin around. He and I spent most of our time on the road together. We were both big fans of the same eighties hardcore punk bands like Black Flag, Minor Threat, Bad Brains, and many others, and bonded over our mutual love of *good* punk rock.

    As much as I liked having Justin around when we were on the road, I started getting really lonely. It was ironic in a lot of ways. Being in a touring band allowed me to meet tons of hot young women, many of whom threw themselves at me. But it was impossible to maintain any sort of meaningful relationship with any of them. I remember trying to have a relationship with someone from Cape Cod I'd met at one of our shows. We'd be out on tour in some far-away state and I'd get a page[1] from her while we

---

[1] Before getting my first cell phone, I always had a pager (aka a beeper). People could page me and it would display a number for me to call them back at when I got to a phone. If they put 911 after the number, it meant it was an emergency. 411

were in the van. By the time I got to a payphone a few hours later, she'd be in bed. Sometimes several days would go by where we kept missing each other like that. Inevitably, her and I broke up – and so did every other woman I tried to have a relationship with while in that band.

After spending a little more than a year rocking out all over the continent, touring really started to take a toll on me. On top of the squabbles with bandmates, the drinking, and the girl problems, there was a lot of pressure from our record label. I joined the band because I wanted to have fun. The label signed the band because they wanted to make money. As time went on, I found myself having less and less fun and feeling more and more suffocated by the business aspect of things. I just wanted to play music. But the label wanted us to sell more merchandise, more records, and what little of our souls we had left. I didn't like it. So I followed the mantra of my teens: when the going gets tough, quit.

I didn't have the guts to face my bandmates and tell them I was out. So I did something I'm apparently known for by quite a few people – I left a note. I've always been a big fan of handwritten notes. Still to this day, anytime someone is kind enough to let me stay in their home, I always leave a thank-you note in a drawer or under a pillow. Why do I do it? I have no fucking idea. But I've been leaving notes since I was a child.

Though I don't remember ever writing them, one of my cousins told me I always left my grandma and grandpa a thank-you note after visiting them in

---

meant they either had or wanted information. Ahhh, the good ol' pager days.

St. Louis as a kid. My father grew up there before joining the military, meeting my mom, and moving to the East Coast where *she* was from. I've told them both several times that raising me in Massachusetts instead of Missouri was the biggest favor they ever did for me. We used to make the twelve-hundred-mile drive to St. Louis every summer to visit my grandparents, aunts, uncles, and cousins. And apparently, every summer I left a thank-you note in my grandma-and-grandpa's house where we always stayed. Years later, a cousin told me that our grandma cherished those notes, keeping every single one of them. I'm glad they made her happy.

    I shouldn't have quit the band by leaving a note. That's the equivalent of breaking up with someone through a text message. It's cowardly and, in a lot of ways, disrespectful. But it's what I did. I'm not proud of it, but it's the truth. I went to the studio when I knew none of my bandmates would be there, packed up all my shit, wrote a short note telling them I was out of the band, left it in the middle of the room with my key, and locked the door on my way out.

"We are all born alone and die alone. The loneliness is definitely part of the journey of life." - Jenova Chen

12. Loneliness

Loneliness is one of the worst feelings a person can experience. Why do you think they stick prisoners in solitary confinement? It's not so they can get some reading done without having to worry about getting shivved. It's not to give them some much-deserved *me* time. It's a punishment – and a cruel one at that. But sadly, it's not at all unusual. Putting prisoners in solitary confinement is common practice because it's one of the meanest, most-torturous things you can do to a person. Nothing breaks a man, woman, or child's spirit like being locked in a cage all alone for days, weeks, months, or even years.

The barbarity of our criminal-justice system aside, loneliness isn't just limited to felons. It's something millions of people feel at least occasionally. And it's something many people with chronic illnesses feel regularly. Loneliness was no stranger to me during my teens and twenties. It's something I felt almost all the time. The situation didn't matter. I could be alone in my bedroom in the middle of the night. I could be among my closest friends at a kick-ass party. I could be with family, coworkers, or whatever girl I happened to be seeing at the time. It didn't matter. Wherever I was, whoever I was with, I felt like my deep-dark secret – my diagnosis – made me different than everyone else. And that led to the loneliness I became so intimately familiar with for the better part of two decades.

In my late teens during the band years, I met a

young woman named Melissa who lived in Stonington, Maine. Melissa invited me to come visit the quaint little island town. To get to Stonington, you have to island hop. From the mainland, you go over a bridge to a large island. From there, you go over another bridge to a smaller island. Then to another and another until you finally arrive on the tiny island of Stonington.

    I liked Melissa and thought she was cool. But she liked *me* in a totally different way. She *liked me*, liked me. Over the years, I've gotten a lot better at understanding how women communicate. Back then, like most guys, I was clueless. I had no idea Melissa liked me *like that*. I'd been a typical, oblivious dude. Looking back, I can now see she threw every nonverbal sign of interest at me a girl possibly can. But they all went right over my head. So I treated her as a friend and nothing more the whole time I was in Stonington. I only stayed for a couple of days. As Melissa and I hugged goodbye, the last thing she did was stick a carefully folded note into one of my pockets.

    When I arrived back home after what should've been a six-hour drive but took almost eight due to a flat tire I got in the hundred-and-five-degree heat, I discovered the note. Now, about twenty-years later, I only remember two things about it. One, Melissa told me that she had feelings for me. I don't recall how she said it exactly, but I remember the sentiment. The other thing I *do* remember word for word. It's a quote she left at the bottom of the note:

    "The worst way to miss someone is to have them sitting right next to you and know you can never have them."

    Those words strummed a chord in my soul

that resonated throughout the entirety of my being. That quote was a metaphor for the nearly constant loneliness I felt from living with Behcet's disease. I knew Melissa didn't mean it that way. She didn't even know I had Behcet's or any illness for that matter. Melissa used the quote to express her unrequited romantic feelings. But it took on a whole different meaning to me.

When you're living with a chronic illness, especially a rare one like Behcet's, you quickly realize that none of your friends, family, coworkers, or acquaintances can possibly understand what it's like to be you. They may mean well. They may try to share in your suffering to make you feel less alone. They may tell you they know what you're going through. But they don't. They couldn't possibly. The only way to know what it's *truly* like is to live through it yourself.

That's why I love the quote Melissa left at the bottom of her handwritten letter. The only difference between what she'd meant and the meaning I'd gotten from the quote lies in its last few words. To Melissa, "never have them" referred to me never sharing the same romantic interest in her that she had in me. But in my interpretation of the quote, "never have them" referred to never having others understand what it's truly like to be me – to really understand what it's like to have a body that's constantly attacking you.

I can't tell you how many well-meaning people I've sat next to yet felt completely alone. Even if it's someone who knew about my illness, one of the rare people I'd talked to about even my most-embarrassing symptoms, they can't *really* know what it's like to experience them. They can't *really* understand what it's like to know they could wake up blind, deaf, or worse on any given day. And in some ways, I'm glad. I don't want the people I care about to know how it feels to have a chronic illness. It's fucking awful.

And it can be wicked lonely.

As early as my late teens, I started thinking about how great it would be to date a woman who also had Behcet's disease. At the time, I'd never really met anyone with the diagnosis, let alone an attractive female around the same age as me. This was long before Facebook groups, Reddit threads, and other places where people with similar diagnoses could hook up. I often fantasized about meeting a young woman with Behcet's at the mall or the grocery store, hitting it off, and jumping into a relationship together – or at least into the sack. That way, I wouldn't have to explain all my painful and embarrassing symptoms, the handful of pills I had to toss down my throat everyday, and everything else that went along with having Behcet's disease. Many of the anxieties that go along with dating wouldn't apply if I could've just met someone with Behcet's.

Too bad, back then, I never did.

It wouldn't be until I was deep into my thirties that I started meeting others with the diagnosis. And that was from online groups, not random encounters at the grocery store. But I still dreamed about hooking up with a woman who also had Behcet's disease for years. All throughout my late teens and twenties, it was one of the most common fantasies I had. I loved the idea of having someone to confide in, someone to share my pain with, someone who knew exactly what I was going through because she was going through it herself. We could be ourselves around each other – both me *and* her – saying whatever was on our minds knowing we wouldn't be judged for it. We could share stories about all the suffering we'd been through, about all the doctors and the meds, and all the other bullshit that goes along with our shared diagnosis. We could explore each other's bodies without the fear of them seeing an old varicose vein or genital scar. We'd understand when the other had to cancel a date because they were too fatigued or in too much pain instead of getting jealous and thinking they were with someone else. We'd no longer each have our own secret to be hidden from the world at all costs. We'd have a shared secret that bonded us closer together than most people ever get to experience. We'd no longer feel constantly alone in the world because we'd have each other.

  It's a nice fantasy, isn't it? Too bad it never happened back in my teens or twenties when I often felt lonely. But I thought about it all the time.

"Doctors are great as long as you don't need them." - Edward E. Rosenbaum

13. Brown

Before leaving the band, the little red bumps on my legs gradually started to return. At first it would just be one or two, here or there. Then it was three or four, here *and* there. By the time I'd quit the band, the fronts of my upper legs were covered in little red bumps just like they had been several years earlier.

Dr. Sack, my rheumatologist, tried to clear up my legs with antibiotics and a topical cream, but neither helped. When those didn't work, in May of 1999 Dr. Sack referred me to nearby Park Dermatology Associates just down the street from his Brockton office. There, I saw a dermatologist named Leonard Horowitz. He was in his early fifties and an accomplished physician with experience treating skin problems of vascular origin like mine. And Dr. Horowitz was board certified in both general *and* pediatric dermatology. Though technically an adult, I was a young one. So it was good to see a dermatologist trained to treat both children and adults.

"Wow," Dr. Horowitz said when I first dropped my jeans so he could examine my upper legs.

"Wow as in this is something so common you see it all the time and can easily treat it?" I asked. "Or wow as in-"

"As in I've never seen such a dense cluster of papulopustular lesions localized to the front of the thighs before," the doctor said.

"That was going to be my second guess."

Dr. Horowitz found my papulopustular

lesions, as he called them, fascinating.[1] He found them *so* interesting they were just too good to keep all to himself. Dr. Horowitz was (and I believe still is) affiliated with Brown University in Providence, RI. If you're not familiar with Brown, it's a private Ivy League university right up there with Harvard, Yale, and Princeton. Currently, Brown University is ranked the fourteenth-best college in the country (out of over two-thousand).[2] Dr. Horowitz asked me if I'd be willing to come to Providence a week later so I could show my legs to some medical students and practicing physicians. It took some convincing but, reluctantly, I agreed. He told me that my participation would help the doctors and students to better treat people like me. And I was under the impression that it'd be an informal thing with just a handful of doctors and students there.

It was not informal, nor were only a few doctors there.

What I'd been invited to was the Brown University Dermatology Clinical Conference held on May 13, 1999. Providence was about forty minutes – with no traffic – from where I lived. Dr. Horowitz asked that I get there nice and early, which meant I had to battle the weekday-morning traffic. I don't recall exactly what time I had to be there. But I *do*

---

[1] I've had doctors refer to the little red bumps on the fronts of my thighs as acne, folliculitis, vascular lesions, papulopustural lesions, and simply as Behcet's sores. Personally, I prefer the term *little red bumps*. Why? Because they look like little red bumps.

[2] 2021 best national university rankings. (n.d.). *U.S. News & World Report.* Retrieved October 6, 2020 from https://www.usnews.com/best-colleges/rankings/national-universities

remember wishing I hadn't agreed to do it the entire drive. With the traffic, it took forever to get to Brown. And once I finally got to the campus, it took forever to find the building I needed to get to. This was still a decade before everyone had GPS. I drove around confused and frustrated trying to get to my destination. Several times, I recall thinking:

Fuck this. I'm going home. What am I even doing here? I shouldn't even be out of bed right now. Yet I'm in a different state, driving around in circles anxiously trying to find one random building among dozens if not hundreds. And for what? So a few med school students can poke me and prod me? Fuck this. I'm out.

Right when I was about to say fuck it and start driving home, I stumbled upon the building I needed to get to. It was a few minutes after Dr. Horowitz asked me to get there. Part of me still wanted to leave. But I hurried into the building and got to where I needed to be. Dr. Horowitz greeted me and brought me into an exam room.

"So how's this going to work?" I asked. "You send in a few doctors and students to look at my legs, ask me a question or two, and then I can go?"

"It might be more than a few," he replied.

"A few what? Doctors and students? Or questions?"

"Both," Dr. Horowitz replied and handed me a johnny.[1] "Take off all your clothes and put this on. Oh, and thank you for agreeing to do this. I know Providence is a bit out of the way for you."

"It's no inconvenience at all," I lied.

---

[1] A johnny is another name for a hospital gown. Sometimes called a johnny gown.

"In a few minutes, the rounds will start."
Rounds? What do you mean rounds?

Before I could ask the doctor what he'd meant, he excused himself and left the room. I put on the johnny and sat on the exam table. My foot wouldn't stop tapping. Having one doctor look at my sore-covered legs, ulcer-covered balls, ulcer-filled mouth, or anything else made me uneasy. The thought of having *rounds* of doctors – whatever that meant – looking at them made the hair on the back of my neck stand straight up.

The exam-room door swung upon. I jumped. Normally, doctors will give a couple of loud knocks on the door before entering to let you know he or she is coming in. I guess that wasn't how they did things at Brown. Dr. Horowitz entered the exam room followed by about a half-dozen wide-eyed medical students. They gathered around me forming a half-circle.

"The subject is an eighteen-year-old male who has a rare form of vasculitis called Behcet's disease," Dr. Horowitz explained to his students. "He was diagnosed at the age of sixteen after several years of unexplained symptoms including..."

I felt like a fucking lab rat. Exposed and vulnerable. There's something dehumanizing about being surrounded by a group of people who are discussing you in the third person. The white lab coats weren't helping either.

"Actually, they started much earlier than that," I said, correcting something the doctor said about one of my symptoms.

"Please refrain from speaking," he replied. "You'll be asked to answer questions soon."

There's something even more dehumanizing

about basically being told to shut the fuck up by the person referring to you in the third person. I'm still not sure why I didn't put my clothes back on, tell every single one of them to suck my ulcer-covered balls, and walk the fuck out of there. That would've totally been something my teenage self would've done. But for whatever reason, I stuck it out.

After Dr. Horowitz gave his little speech about the subject – I mean his speech about *me* – he opened up the floor to questions. Several med students asked away. Some of their questions were quite good. Some of them even gave me insights into my illness that I hadn't considered. When our allotted time was up, they left the exam room and were replaced by another group of students. Then another. And another.

I don't remember how many different groups of med students I saw that morning, but it was several. I was at Brown for hours. After the first group, it wasn't so bad. In some ways, I actually kind of liked it. There I was, an eighteen-year-old kid educating third-and-forth-year medical students about a disease they knew nothing about. That would be the beginning of my doctor-educating career. Since Behcet's is so rare, most doctors don't know shit about the disease. I've had to educate many of the doctors I've been to over the years about the specifics of Behcet's. It gives me a little sliver of satisfaction. I do like to teach – almost as much as I like to learn. But don't get me wrong: I wish I didn't have to teach them anything. I'd definitely prefer it if medical professionals were better educated about Behcet's.

Word must've traveled the Brown campus that morning about the dude with zit-covered legs and big ulcers in his mouth and on his balls. Because after the med students were done, groups of licensed physicians in several different specialties came into the exam room. They weren't nearly as fun as the students. One of the doctors asked if he could snap a few photos of my legs for an upcoming dermatology textbook he was editing. He assured me my face wouldn't be in it, so I said it'd be fine.

Snap. Snap.

"This is great," Shutterbug MD said as he photographed my legs. "I've never seen clusters this dense on the legs before."

Snap.

"What did I tell you?" Dr. Horowitz replied to his colleague.

Snap. Snap, snap, snap.

Going to Brown University and being a lab rat was an interesting experience. In some ways it made me feel special. I got to educate doctors about a disease so rare they might not ever get to see another case in their entire medical careers. It was awkward and embarrassing at times, but I got through it. Would I ever agree to do something like that again? Hell no. But I'm glad I had the experience.

I don't remember what Dr. Horowitz put me on for the little red bumps on my legs. I'm not even sure if I ever saw him again after the conference in Providence. I don't recall ever seeing him again. And if I did, I have no record of it. What I *do* recall is the little red bumps on my legs going away a few months later. Unfortunately, they didn't go *away*, away. They just moved to my chest.

"The person who takes medicine must recover twice, once from the disease and once from the medicine." - William Osler, MD

14. Sex & Drugs

After I'd been kicked out my first band, I still spent a lot of time down at River's Edge Studio. After quitting the second band, I more or less stopped hanging out there entirely. My experience being on the road, following a grueling touring schedule, being away from the people I cared about, having to deal with our record label, getting exposed the super-shady business side of the music industry, and constantly having access to free drugs and alcohol really made me question things. It all forced me to reevaluate what I wanted in life. Before then it was clear: I wanted to be a rockstar. That was my dream all throughout my teens. But after voluntarily leaving the nationally-touring band, I seriously started to rethink those rockstar dreams.

Eventually, I made the decision to never mix my love of playing music with my disgust of the music industry. In other words, music would forever remain a hobby and never my source of income. Music was sacred to me. It still is. I didn't want to pollute my love of music with the necessary nastiness that goes along with being successful in the music industry. It really should be called the *image industry*. During my band years, I saw so many amazing bands get ignored by major labels because they didn't fit the image those labels were looking for. And I also saw a lot of shitty bands get signed to million-dollar deals. Limp Bizkit comes to mind. When they got signed to Interscope, there were ten other bands playing the same style of music that were twenty times more talented. But they didn't have the look and the connections that Fred Durst and the boys did. Same thing with Godsmack. They weren't even a real band for fuck's sake: they were an Alice In Chains cover band! But they had the look and the connections to get signed. That's the way it works in the music industry. Image trumps music and has for a long time. I don't give a fuck about image. I think the music should speak for itself. So I abandoned my rockstar dreams and decided to forever keep music as a hobby and not a job.

    I had a lot of free time after I quit the band. My friend Sarah and I got full-time jobs together doing data entry for a women's clothing store. Neither of us particularly liked working there but it paid well. We got out at four everyday so, with no band practice to get to, my evenings and weekends were free.

    Even though my band days were behind me, I still had a lot of friends in bands and enjoyed going to shows. My favorite band to watch practice was a super-heavy-metal band that practiced down The Cape.[1] Herbie, the drummer from my first band, played for them. Every weekend I'd head down to Falmouth with my bottle of Vicodin ES to watch them practice. They were always great and full of energy. The house they practiced at belonged to the guitar-player's-cousin's mother. She was from Ireland and had a thick Gaelic accent. I don't think I ever saw her sober. Not once. It didn't matter what time of day it was – first thing in the morning, middle of the day, late at night – she was always drinking. But I really didn't see very much of her at all. She spent most of

---

[1] Cape Cod, Massachusetts.

her time at her boyfriend's house on the other side of town. Even when she was around, she didn't care who was at her house, what they were doing, or how much noise they were making. It made for the perfect hangout spot.

One Saturday after Herbie's band finished their afternoon practice session, he and I drove an hour to Brockton for what was supposed to be an awesome concert. When we got there, we found out that it had been canceled. The venue was locked and there was no one there except for two cute young women sitting outside on the sidewalk. They didn't know the show had been canceled either and got dropped off there a little earlier. As it turned out, Herbie knew both of them. And one of them knew *me*. She didn't know me personally, but she knew *of* me from the time I'd spent in my last band.

The four of us went back to Falmouth. Me and Stephanie, the gorgeous young woman who'd known me by reputation, hit it off immediately. The two of us spent the night together on the couch cuddling, kissing, and talking. That would be the beginning of a tumultuous two-year relationship with a woman I definitely didn't deserve. Between my unpredictable behavior and all the lies I threw at her to hide the fact that I had a horrible disease, I was a lousy boyfriend.

Some of the worst genital ulcers I've ever had were during the two years Stephanie and I spent together. Not only were they incredibly painful, the ulcers made it nearly impossible to have a normal sex life. When they were really bad, I didn't want Stephanie going anywhere near my crotch. I was always coming up with excuses to keep my super-hot girlfriend away from there. And when I say *super hot*, that's not just my opinion. Stephanie was an award-winning fashion model. Most guys would've killed just to be in her presence. I was the envy of all my male friends – a few female friends, too. Yet I was always coming up with reasons to keep Stephanie away from me.

In hindsight, I think my unpredictable behavior made Stephanie like me even more. I was nineteen when we met and she was eighteen-months younger than me. Though I'd lost my virginity three-years earlier and already had several girlfriends, Stephanie was still a virgin and I was her first real boyfriend. I sent that poor girl on an emotional rollercoaster ride that probably made her feel incredibly insecure. As women get older, they often learn to avoid relationships like that. They learn to avoid guys like nineteen-year-old me. But for an innocent young woman like Stephanie, all the craziness can be exciting and even addicting.

Speaking of which, by the time her and I'd met, my pain-pill addiction was in full swing. Sometimes when I ran out of pills, I'd have Stephanie help me get more. As if regularly lying to her wasn't bad enough, I also turned her into an accomplice to my raging opioid addiction. A few months after we got together, Stephanie's father had a minor heart attack. The doctors prescribed him Vicodin (regular strength, not the extra-strength ones like I was prescribed) and Valium, neither of which he took very often and both sat unprotected in a cabinet above the kitchen sink. On more than one occasion, I had Stephanie steal some for me.

"Thanks, babe," I said as Stephanie placed three Vicodin in my sweaty, shaky hand from the passenger seat of my Nissan Sentra.

"You're welcome, baby," she replied with a

smile. "I hate to see you like this. I'd do anything to make you feel better."

"I know. You're the best," I said, throwing all three pills down my throat, followed by a few gulps of Mountain Dew.

"I wish we could spend some time together tonight," Stephanie said, taking my clammy hand into one of hers.

"I know. Me too. But my friends are expecting me."

"I know they are," Stephanie replied, doing the best she could to hide her disappointment. "I understand. Can we spend some time together tomorrow?"

"We'll see. I probably still won't be feeling well. Maybe you can grab a few more Vikes for me."

"I really shouldn't. I know my father doesn't take them very often but I don't want them to all be gone in case he needs them."

"Yeah, I understand," I replied, slowly pulling my hand away. "I probably won't be around tomorrow then. I'll be busy trying to get my hands on some more Vikes so I don't feel so shitty."

Stephanie tilted her head slightly to the side. With wide, puppy-dog eyes, she looked at me and smiled. The girl absolutely adored me and I treated her like garbage.

"Maybe I can grab you just a couple more pills tomorrow," she said.

"I'll need at least three to feel decent."

"Okay," Stephanie replied. "I can do that. I can get three for you tomorrow. So you'll come over and spend time with me?"

"Sure," I answered and smiled, taking her hand once again. "For a little while at least. But right now, I have to get going. My friends are expecting me."

Stephanie flashed her big, beautiful smile. We kissed for a few minutes in her parents' driveway before saying goodbye. She got out of my car and I watched Stephanie's perfect ass sway from side to side as she walked back to the house.

I was a lousy boyfriend. Stephanie was as sweet as she was sexy, but I didn't fully appreciate what an amazing young woman she was at the time. I put everything before her: my pills, my friends, my hobbies, and myself. All she wanted to do was spend time with me. Don't get me wrong: I loved spending time with Stephanie, too – but only after popping a handful of pills or downing a half-bottle of liquor. Granted, I was legitimately in pain almost every day. And I was clearly depressed and overflowing with anxiety. The pills and alcohol gave me enough relief from those things that I could enjoy social interaction. But none of that excuses the way I treated Stephanie. It explains it, but it doesn't excuse it.

In addition to the genital and oral ulcers, I had some other skin issues during the two years we were together. Just like the little red bumps that had returned to my upper legs a few months *before* meeting Stephanie, I started getting them on my chest a few months *after* meeting her. At first, there were just a few of them. But over the course of a couple months, my entire upper chest became covered. Each of my pecs had dozens, maybe hundreds of red bumps all over them. Some of them had little whiteheads but most of them didn't. Some of them hurt but, fortunately, most did not. The one thing they all *did* have in common was that they looked ugly and caused me a lot of anxiety.

My chest was at its worst in the summer of 2000. I didn't have an air conditioner where I was living so I often went shirtless. When Stephanie was over, all I could think about was how bad I looked. She never said anything about the bumps and often ran her soft, manicured hands all over my chest. I doubt Stephanie thought it was anything more than normal guy acne. But I always worried she'd figure out there was something seriously wrong with me. That fear loomed over our entire relationship.

Not only did the visible manifestations of Behcet's not lead Stephanie to thinking something was wrong with me, in some cases they actually made her find me more attractive. The blood clots I'd had over a year before meeting Stephanie caused a large vein to rise to the surface of my abdomen. Now I've got several varicose veins on my abs and all over both legs. But at the time there was just that one. The twisty vein ran from the left side of the top of my abs down to my crotch. On several occasions, Stephanie told me that she found the vein to be incredibly sexy. She even used to drag her tongue over it when she was working her way down to that area.

Over the past twenty years since Stephanie and I were together, I've had several other women tell me that they find my varicose veins sexy. But the compliments haven't been limited to women. I've had a number of guys comment on how they wish they had veins like that. Vascularity is generally an indicator of health. Lots of women find vascularity to be sexy and lots of guys want their veins to be visible. I've always been very vascular. The veins in my forearms and the one on each bicep[1] have been

---

[1] The cephalic vein, for you A&P nerds out there.

clearly visible for as long as I can remember. Those I like. But I've always hated the varicose veins in my legs and abs from all the clots. But women can't seem to get enough of them.

    I never told Stephanie that the vein she'd been so fond of looked like that because I had a rare, chronic disease. If I had, I bet she no longer would've found it attractive. Over the years, I've told the truth to a couple of the women I've dated who said they found one or more of my varicose veins sexy. And whenever I have, the compliments about how sexy they are usually seem to stop. While I'm always upfront about having Behcet's disease now, there are still some things that I don't bring up unless directly asked. My varicose veins are one of those things.

    Stephanie was such a sweetheart. She thought she was helping her boyfriend. But in reality she was just enabling me. To make extra money, Stephanie would sometimes babysit. And whenever she could, she'd invite me over to come hang out with her. As soon as I got to wherever she was babysitting, the first chance I got I'd rummage through all the bathroom and kitchen cabinets looking for pills. You'd be surprised how many people have pain pills just lying around.

    I don't know how I managed to not drive Stephanie away with all that craziness. But she stayed with me for almost two years. It was the last few months of our relationship that finally drove her away. But not because of my drinking, drug use, lies, or strange behavior. It was because, for the first time in years, I got clean and sober.

"So many good things come in pairs like ears, socks, and panda bears. But, best of all are the set of twins with extra laughter, double grins." - Anonymous

15. Broken

I remember the first time I thought about killing myself. I was in early middle school. Even though I was still years away from a diagnosis, my body was regularly kicking my ass. I thought to myself, *I would rather not exist at all than be in pain all the time.*

When I was thirteen, the biggest hero I'd ever had committed suicide. I'll never forget how I found out. I was at home and it was a little before supper time. My mother was in the kitchen cooking and my father was watching the news in the living room. I came out of my room to see how much longer until dinner. My dad got up to do the same thing and gave me the news as he walked into the kitchen.

"You hear? Your hero's dead," he said matter-of-factly with a shit-eating grin on his face.

"What?" I asked.

"Cobain or whatever his name is. He killed himself."

My dad seemed amused by the news. I was devastated. Like so many others of my generation, Kurt's lyrics spoke to me. He was in pain, just like me.

For the next couple weeks, Kurt's suicide was all anyone could talk about. I kept hearing things like:

"What a waste of talent."

"What a fool. He had it all."

"Why would he do such a thing?"

But my opinion was different. I couldn't help

but think, *I get it*.

Being in pain sucks. Add depression, anxiety, and drugs into the mix and it's the recipe for a miserable existence. That's how I felt almost all the time: miserable. I'd be lying if I said there weren't occasional pockets of fun and joy in there, but most of my adolescence was awful.

Suicide was something I thought about a lot once I got into my teens. By the time I was in my late teens, I thought about it daily. I was already in pain, depressed, and anxious. And my growing pill-and-alcohol addictions just threw gas on the already brightly burning fire. The more I thought about suicide, the more attractive the idea got.

Shortly after becoming and adult, I had to stop going to the pediatrician I'd seen all throughout childhood and adolescence. My new primary care physician was an internist named Richard Gross. He was a soft-spoken man about fifty-years-old with glasses and a mostly full head of white hair. While I did like his laid-back demeanor and pleasant personality, I questioned some of the medical decisions Dr. Gross made over the years he was my PCP. One of his earliest decisions is one I still question to this day.

Dr. Gross wasn't just *my* primary care physician. He was also my father's and, for a while, my mother's as well. When I was twenty, my dad told Dr. Gross I was severely depressed and needed to go on an antidepressant. Apparently, Dr. Gross agreed. Because the next time I saw him, he put me on Prozac.

One cold, winter night, I went out with Stephanie, my friend Chris, and some girl he had with him. Stephanie and I were about a year and a half into our relationship at that point. We all went to the theater to see a movie: Dungeons and Dragons. Chris and I used to play D&D in middle school, but I gave it up when I discovered weed, wine, and women. Speaking of wine, I managed to talk Stephanie into grabbing a big bottle of wine and some gin from her parents' liquor cabinet for us. And by *us*, I mostly meant *me*. Stephanie and the other girl took a couple of small sips, but I ended up drinking most of the booze myself.

  The movie sucked. It sucked so badly that, halfway through, I stumbled out of the theater and demanded a refund for the four of us. Then after getting the refund, my drunk ass stumbled back into the theater and finished watching the movie with the others. When it was over, Chris brought us all home.

  I don't remember exactly what happened that night, but I do remember bits and pieces of it. Once I got home, I went up to my room. In spite of having a good night with a friend and my girlfriend, I quickly became extremely depressed. I was incredibly drunk and should've just tried to go to sleep. But that's not what I did.

  I remember calling Stephanie a few times. It was after midnight. I wanted to say goodbye to her but never got the chance.

  "Hello?" Stephanie's father answered.

  "H... Hi," I replied, unsuccessfully trying not to sound too shitfaced. "Can I t...talk please with Steph, puhleeese?"

  "Do you realize what time it is?" he asked in his deep, booming voice.

  "I know I'm... I know it's late. But I just need..."

  "You can talk to my daughter in the morning.

Do not call here this late again."

Click.

    I'm not sure how many times I tried calling Stephanie that night but it was more than once. Overcome with guilt, shame, embarrassment, anxiety, depression, and just about every other negative emotion I can think of, I scribbled a suicide note on a piece of paper. Then, using a razor blade, I started slashing away at my wrists.

    With my eyes filled with tears, I made close to a dozen cuts. Half the tears were of joy, the others of sorrow. Knowing my suffering would soon be over brought a wave of immense happiness. But it was mixed with the sadness of leaving behind so many people I cared about, as well as an endlessly interesting world I'd only begun to explore. I watched the blood drip from my arms, adding even more color to the off-white carpet I'd stained a million times before. Three years worth of spilled grape juice, fruit punch, Mountain Dew, and candle wax decorated the carpet, most of it between the door and my nightstand. The bright-red blood stains were dead in the center of the room, just as I imagined my body would soon be.

    But as it turns out, it's a lot harder to kill yourself than you might think – especially when you're rip-roaring drunk.

    What *isn't* hard is waking up your entire family while *trying* to kill yourself. Hearing me stumbling around, crying, and probably making all sorts of other noises, my father woke up and came into my room. I don't actually remember anything at this point, but my brother tells me that dad started yelling and freaking out, which I don't doubt. He was a frequent yeller and freaker-outer. My brother's a night owl like me and was awake in his room down the hall. Hearing all the yelling, both my brother and mother came running into my room to see what all the commotion was. They called 911 and a few minutes later my room was filled with cops and paramedics.

It's funny how things work out sometimes. When sober, I knew you had to run the blade up your arm to kill yourself. But when I was sober, I didn't have the balls to kill myself. When I was drunk, I did have the balls. But in my inebriated state, I'd somehow managed to forget the right way to do it and started slicing away at my arms from left to right, not top to bottom. The result was not the end to my suffering I'd hoped for. The result was about a dozen superficial cuts, a couple of serious cuts that required stitches, and a week-long trip to the psych hospital. Ultimately, all I did was *add* to my suffering.

At the time, no one – myself included – even considered that going on Prozac just a month or two earlier might've played a role in my suicide attempt. But years later, as more and more studies showed that antidepressant use in teens and young adults dramatically increased suicide risk,[1] I did start to consider it. Could the Prozac have contributed to my suicide attempt? There's no way to prove it, but the timing is awfully suspicious. But if it did play a role – even a large role – the Prozac didn't act alone. I'd been suicidal for years. Pain pills and alcohol were definitely part of the equation. And I'd been on another prescription drug that likely played a much bigger role than the Prozac, Vicodin, and alcohol

---

[1] The association between suicidality and Prozac in patients my age was known at the time Dr. Gross prescribed it to me. I don't know if he was aware of this correlation – but he should've been.

combined: prednisone. After being on a high dose of prednisone for many months, coming off it led to uncontrollable mood swings, panic attacks, and several varieties of physical discomfort. If a single drug was responsible for my suicide attempt, it would've been prednisone, not Prozac. That being said, the Prozac definitely didn't help. It had no noticeable effect on my mood and came with a few minor-but-annoying side effects.

The paramedics brought me to Morton Hospital where a doctor stitched up my wrists. They had me talk to a social worker, who ordered me to be sent to a psychiatric hospital with a dual-diagnosis unit. These specialized units are for patients with both mental health and substance abuse issues. A while after talking to the social worker, an ambulance arrived and took me to Arbor-Fuller Hospital in Attleboro about forty-five minutes away.

As the alcohol slowly wore off, the reality of my situation gradually crept in. Looking down at my bandaged arms made me want to cry. The paramedic in the back with me did his best to make me feel better, but I could tell by the look on his face that he knew I was in need of some serious help. We got to the psych hospital and they wheeled me in on the stretcher. My anxiety doubled with every passing second as we approached the dual-diagnosis unit.

What are people going to think? What are they going to say? How long am I going to be stuck here for?

These and a million other questions filled my head. The paramedics wheeled me into the unit that would be my home for who-knew-how-long. As we approached the check-in area, my anxiety started bordering on panic. A cute blond girl about my age walked up to me while I was still on the stretcher. I could feel my heart beating in the back of my throat as she approached me. But then, with just three simple words, she made every last drop of my anxiety evaporate in an instant.

"Look!" the girl said, holding up two bandaged wrists of her own. "We're twins!"

I don't think I said anything, but I'm sure I smiled – at least a little bit. She smiled back and I couldn't help but notice that one of her top front teeth was missing.

"I'm Kady," the thin, blond girl said. "It's spelled K-A-D-Y, but it's pronounced just like Katie."

"Hi Kady," I replied. "I'm Ellis. It's nice to meet you."

"Nice to meet you, too," she said and shook my hand, our bandaged wrists lightly brushing against each other.

Kady and I quickly became friends. She'd been struggling with opioids, alcohol, depression, and anxiety, too. We often took our cigarette breaks together whenever possible. On one of those first smoke breaks, Kady told me her tooth had recently been kicked out by a guy who raped her. She didn't seem phased by it and told the story with little emotion. I think it bothered me more than it did her. Kady and I had a lot of great conversations, but it was those first few words she'd said to me when the paramedics wheeled me in that I'll never forget. They really put me at ease and made me think that maybe, just maybe things were going to be alright.

The psych hospital really wasn't all that bad. I got to meet some really interesting people and it gave me some much-needed time away from the drudgery of everyday life. The only things that sucked were that I didn't have any cigarettes and I was in pain from the sores in my mouth. Fortunately, within twenty-four hours of being admitted, I managed to solve both problems. I called Stephanie and had her bring me a couple packs of Marlboro Reds and a lighter. One pack, I had her give to a woman working on the dual-diagnosis unit. The staff held onto our cigarettes, only giving them out at certain times. The other pack along with the lighter, I had her sneak in to me. We were only allowed maybe five or six cigarette breaks a day and I was used to smoking a lot more than that.

    I attacked my opioid problem on two fronts. First, I talked to the psychiatrist assigned to me. I'd been to enough doctors to know what to say to get what I wanted. I played up the Behcet's angle and convinced her to prescribe me some Percocet. The order was written as one every six hours. My opioid tolerance was high from being on Vicodin ES for so long and I quickly learned that one Perc did nothing for my pain. So I started cheeking them and taking two at a time before dinner so I could eat mostly pain free.

    On the other opioid front was Kady. She didn't use them to treat physical pain like I primarily did. Kady used them to self-medicate her emotional pain, as many people do. That was just a bonus for me. I took them to relieve the many varieties of bodily pain the Behcet's caused but certainly enjoyed the effect they had on my mood, as well. Kady came up with a plan to have someone sneak her in some heroin and was kind enough to include me in the reward, even though she took all the risk.

    The dual-diagnosis unit was a locked unit, but we were allowed to have visitors. Kady had someone come bring her a few bags of heroin, assuring the guy she had the money to pay him. They went into the visitation room and talked for a few minutes. She slid him a sealed envelope across the table and he handed her the drugs under it. I just happened to be passing by the visitation room at the time and saw the scruffy-looking dude about to open the envelope.

"Don't open it here!" I heard Kady say as I was passing by the visitation-room door which was open just a crack. "If they see you counting money, we'll both get in lots of trouble. You can count it when you get outside. Don't worry. It's all there."

The guy eyed Kady for a moment, then slipped the envelope into his pocket. They talked for another minute and then she asked one of the staff to unlock the door to let him off the unit.

"Don't let him back in here," she told the staff as soon as he was gone. "He threatened me. Don't let him or anyone else in here to see me other than my parents unless I say it's okay."

Kady disappeared into her room for a few minutes, then came out with constricted pupils and a big, goofy smile on her face. We went down the hall, made sure we were out of sight of any hospital staff, and had a seat. She handed me a little bag of brownish-white powder.

"Let me know what you think," Kady said, speaking slower than usual. "It's not the best I've ever had, but it's good."

"I will," I replied. "Thank you so much. I don't have any way to repay you, but I'll throw you a couple of cigarettes."

"Don't even worry about it," she said with a mischievous grin. "It didn't cost me anything."

"Then what was in the envelope?" I asked.

"Clippings from today's newspaper."

I looked at Kady for a moment to try to gauge whether or not she was telling the truth. There was no doubt in my mind: she was. At the same time, we both burst out in laughter.

"You're fucking crazy," I said, still laughing.

"Says the dude who's in a mental hospital," she replied smirkin' it up.

We both laughed our asses off. Kady made my stay at Arbor-Fuller Hospital more than tolerable – she made it almost enjoyable. The next morning, her and I were the last two to show up for the first group of the day. I guarantee we slept better than any of the other patients that night. Heroin's good for that. It's also really bad for a lot of things. But it's definitely good for pain and sleep.

I was only at Arbor-Fuller for about a week before being discharged. From there, I was sent to Gosnold Treatment Center, a rehab facility down in Falmouth. Kady was sad I'd be leaving before her but we promised to keep in touch and get together at some point. I only talked to her one more time after that, my first night in rehab. When I finally got home from there, I tried calling Kady twice. Both times, her parents answered the phone. The first time it was her mom. Then a few days later, her dad.

"Hi, is Kady there?" I asked.

"She's not taking any calls for a long, long time," he said.

"Please," I replied. "I just want to talk to her for a minute."

"Kady will not be associating with anyone that she knows anymore."

"You don't understand. We met in Arbor-Fuller. I'm not someone from the street that she's used with. I just got out of rehab myself. I'm clean."

"I've made myself clear. Do not call here or make any attempt at contacting my daughter again."

"But if you'd just-"

Click.

I always wondered what happened to Kady. For years, I assumed the worst. When I knew her, Kady's addiction was strong and her behavior was reckless. I still can't believe she had the balls to rip off the drug dealer the way she did. I thought for sure something bad probably happened to Kady, as was so often the case with other friends who had serious addictions.

But imagine my surprise when I found her on Facebook about a year ago when I was writing the first draft of this book. I was reflecting on the week we'd spent together at Arbor-Fuller almost two-decades earlier and decided to look her up. I really didn't expect to find her. For years I figured she'd passed away. Kady's addiction was stronger than many of the addicts I knew who *did* pass. But sure enough, I found Kady on Facebook and sent her a friend request. She accepted it and I wrote her a long message thanking her for making my experience at Arbor-Fuller less horrible than it could've been. We messaged back and forth, catching up on the last twenty years. After her hospital stay, Kady struggled for a few more years. But eventually she got clean and started a new life for herself. She's doing well now and I couldn't be happier for her. I thought for sure she was dead. But somehow she made it. Somehow her story has a happy ending, just like mine. I guess I shouldn't be too surprised, though. After all, we are – or at least *were*, once upon a time – twins.

"Drugs made me feel more normal." - Carrie Fisher

16. Fixed

I spent a few weeks in rehab down The Cape before they let me go home. It was awful. Not only would they not prescribe me any opioids for the legitimate pain I was in, they wouldn't even let us have caffeine.

A lot of doctors don't think of fatigue as a primary symptom of Behcet's disease – if they think about Behcet's at all. Uveitis, genital and oral ulcers, blood clots, and the other visible symptoms get all the attention. But brain fog and excessive tiredness seem to go hand-in-hand with Behcet's for a lot of patients. I spent a lot of time in bed while I was in rehab. There wasn't anyone there I connected with like I had with Kady on the dual-diagnosis unit at Arbor-Fuller. Out of the entire time I was at Gosnold, I can only recall one positive memory from the whole experience. It wasn't even really positive – just funny.

My roommate was an asshole. He was a loud, cocky, entitled, womanizing piece of shit who was detoxing from alcohol. The doctors had him on Librium[1] and it knocked him out pretty hard. One afternoon, I got woken up from a nap by the sound of water splashing. I looked over at my dickhead roommate and saw him lying butt-naked in bed on his back, his small-but-erect cock pointing straight up at the ceiling. He was pissing several feet into the air like a fountain and it was splashing back down all

---

[1] Librium (chlordiazepoxide) is a benzodiazepine, the same class of drugs as Xanax, Ativan, Klonopin, and many others. It's used to treat anxiety, insomnia, and alcohol withdrawal syndrome.

over his body. It was fucking hilarious.

Although the doctors at the rehab wouldn't prescribe me anything stronger than ibuprofen for my pain, they did refer me to a pain-management clinic at Brigham and Women's Hospital in Boston as part of my aftercare plan. They also referred me to a psychiatrist and a therapist.

I don't remember the doctor's name that I saw at the pain management clinic, just that he was an exceptionally good-looking man with a full head of white hair and a charming personality. He recognized that I was in a lot of pain and needed something for it. But the doctor thought it'd be best if I stopped taking Vicodin since it contains a lot of acetaminophen, especially the extra-strength variety I'd been on for several years at that point. The first thing he prescribed me was tramadol, a fully-synthetic opioid that had recently been approved by the FDA. It barely took the edge off.

When I took the T[2] into Boston to see the pain management doctor again a month later, he wrote me a prescription for another fully-synthetic opioid: methadone. I'd heard about its use in getting people off heroin but I didn't know it was also used for pain. I was pleasantly surprised by how well it worked. Not only did it make my pain more manageable, it did so without causing the highs and lows that Vicodin did. Methadone has a much longer half-life than hydrocodone,[3] the semi-synthetic opioid in Vicodin,

---

[2]   The T is what we call the MBTA (Massachusetts Bay Transportation Authority). It's Boston's subway and commuter rail system.

[3]   A drug's half life is the amount of time it takes for your body to eliminate half of it from your system. Hydrocodone (Vicodin) has a half life of about 4 hours. Methadone has an

and its effects last considerably longer. With just one or two doses a day, I'd get round-the-clock relief from the pain I was in.

Being on methadone also helped me to stay away from alcohol for a while. After leaving rehab, I decided to do my best to stay away from booze. The methadone helped to ease my anxiety and depression a little bit. Not completely, but it definitely took the edge off.

The months following my release from rehab were quite boring. No going out and getting shitfaced all the time. No begging Stephanie to steal drugs and alcohol from her parents for me. I made a real effort to be a better boyfriend to her during those months – and I was. Unfortunately, it wasn't the sober, better me that Stephanie had fallen in love with almost two years earlier. She fell for the crazy, manipulative, pill-popping, booze-guzzling, emotional-train-wreck me. When I came out of rehab, that guy was gone – for a while, at least.

A few months into my sobriety, Stephanie left me for another guy. I was hurt at the time and I called her a bunch of names I still regret to this day. But I met a young woman named Caitlin from down The Cape soon after who helped me to quickly get over Stephanie. Interestingly enough, Caitlin ended up leaving me a few months later for the *exact opposite* reason. I had been sober when Caitlin and I met but started drinking and dabbling with drugs again a month or two into our relationship. She liked the sober me and my drug and alcohol use scared her away. But Caitlin and I had a few good months together and she made getting over Stephanie a lot

---

average half life of about 22 hours.

easier than it would've been otherwise.

The therapist that the rehab referred me to wasn't much help. He was a nice-enough guy, a middle-aged social worker named Bob who worked for Community Counseling of Bristol County (CCBC). But he seemed to be just as depressed as me – maybe even more so. Though I didn't know him at the time, Bob lived just two houses down from me for a few years when I was a kid. Small world. The psychiatric nurse I was referred to, however, *was* helpful.

After getting released from Gosnold, I moved back in with my parents for a while. One of the conditions they set for living with them was that I had to go to college. I didn't want to live with them *or* go to college. But at the time I didn't have much of a choice. So I enrolled at Bristol Community College (BCC), a small two-year state school in Fall River about thirty-minutes away.

I'd always done well in school as a kid. It wasn't until high school that my grades started slipping. But it wasn't because I struggled with the material. I just thought it was pointless to learn a bunch of stuff I knew I wasn't going to ever use. But my first couple semesters at BCC, I *did* struggle. I was put on academic probation and almost flunked out of community college. It was embarrassing. My brain was often foggy and, even when it wasn't, I usually had trouble focusing. It's impossible to know what caused those symptoms. It could've been one of the after-effects of being on long-term, high-dose prednisone in my late teens. It could've been due to some sort of inflammation in the brain caused by the Behcet's. It could've been a combination of those things. Or it could've been due to something else altogether. Who knows.

There's no question being on high-dose prednisone – or more accurately, *coming off* high-dose prednisone – fucked me up. I'm sure it contributed to my depression and anxiety. But to what degree it played in my brain fog is unclear. What *is* clear is the stretch marks it left all over my ass. The prednisone caused me to quickly gain a lot of weight, almost all of it in my belly and butt. When I came off the prednisone, just as quickly as I'd gained it, I lost the extra weight. I don't have any stretch marks on my belly, but my butt is covered with them. They used to make me extremely self-conscious which is kind of ridiculous. It's not like they're somewhere a lot of people would see them. Very few people had the privilege of seeing my pale, stretch-mark-covered ass during my late teens and early twenties. Now the stretch marks don't bother me at all. Now I'm happy to show off my pale, stretch-mark-covered caboose to anyone who wants to see it.

The psychiatric nurse I began seeing who also worked at CCBC first put me on Wellbutrin, which didn't do anything for me. She also tried a couple of antidepressants. Aside from a few minor, annoying side effects, they didn't help my mood, energy levels, or brain fog either. Then she put me on Concerta, a time-released form of methylphenidate that had just recently been approved by the FDA.[2] I took it for a couple months but it didn't seem to do much. Then she prescribed Dexedrine, which was a game changer.

I went from almost flunking out of community

---

[2] Methylphenidate is the generic name for Ritalin, the well-known ADHD medication. Concerta is basically time-released Ritalin and became available in 2000 after gaining FDA approval that year.

college to breezing through the next two years with straight As. The Dexedrine gave me the energy and focus needed to excel in school. After getting my associates degree, I transferred to Bridgewater State College (now University), another state school. Though I didn't really like going to community college, I *did* like Bridgewater. I double-majored in psychology and philosophy, two subjects I'd been passionate about since my mid-teens. The courses were a lot more challenging than the ones at community college, which I liked. Being on Dexedrine, I was easily able to handle four-to-five classes each semester. Without them, it would've been a struggle just to pass one.

While still going to community college, I switched from seeing a psychiatric nurse to seeing an actual psychiatrist at CCBC named Dr. Karlin. He was and remains to this day the most competent, compassionate, and all-around-best mental-health provider I've ever met. The mental health field is filled with well-intentioned people, but most of them don't really know what they're doing. I say this not only as a patient who has been to several therapists and psychiatrists, but also as someone who went to school for clinical psychology and worked in the mental health field for over fifteen years. I've worked with dozens – maybe hundreds – of therapists, psychologists, psychiatrists, psychiatric nurses, and other mental health professionals. Most of them are pretty useless. Many of them are more fucked up than their patients/clients. That's what attracts them to the mental-health field in the first place. They're either fucked up themselves or were close to someone who was growing up. That's why they get into the field: they want to understand what's wrong with themselves and to help others who are similarly fucked up. Sadly, few mental-health professionals actually make any meaningful difference in their patients'/clients' lives. But for what it's worth (which is basically nothing if you're a patient/client), most of them mean well and really do *want* to help.

Dr. Karlin switched me from Dexedrine to a similar-but-slightly-different drug which helped with the fatigue and brain fog even more. He also put me on a few other psych meds to help with my depression, anxiety, and sleep. I called it The Magic Combo. Those meds had me feeling decent most of the time which was something I hadn't consistently felt in over a decade.

When you're used to feeling like shit all the time, feeling decent is almost euphoric. I still had a negative outlook on life, but the day-to-day drudgery seemed less cumbersome. When simply getting through the day is a monumental task in and of itself, it's hard to get anything else done. But feeling decent allowed me to actually accomplish stuff. In addition to going to college full time, I was able to work. I had a series of mostly part-time jobs that I mostly full-time hated. But I needed money and they paid for my gas, food, rent, and helped me build up a respectable CD[1] collection.

The summer after graduating from BCC but before starting at BSC that fall, I trained for a job I thought I'd actually like. During the summer of 2003 when I turned twenty-three, I got certified as an

---

[1] Compact Disc (CD). They were how we used to buy and listen to music before mp3s, YouTube, Spotify, and other online services popped up. CDs became popular in the late 80s and early 90s and were preferred over cassettes and vinyl by most people.

Emergency Medical Technician (EMT). Those are the guys trained in emergency medicine who show up in an ambulance when you call 911. EMTs respond to car accidents, gunshot wounds, stabbings, drug overdoses – *lots* of drug overdoses – heart attacks, strokes, severe allergic reactions, and other medical and psychiatric emergencies. EMT training was challenging, but I loved it. As soon as I got certified by the state, I began applying for EMT jobs.

By the time I transferred to Bridgewater State College, the Behcet's was mostly in remission. I hadn't had any serious symptoms like uveitis or blood clots since my teens. And the ulcers in my mouth and on my balls gradually got less and less frequent until they stopped entirely. I eventually tapered off methadone and stopped going to the pain management clinic. Aside from a couple of psych meds, I wasn't taking any other prescription drugs. No immunosuppressants, no corticosteroids, no painkillers, nothing. Overall, my heath – both physical and mental – was better than it had been in over a decade.

Unfortunately, it wouldn't stay that way for very long.

"Maybe self-improvement isn't the answer. Maybe self-destruction is the answer." - Tyler Durden (from Fight Club by Chuck Palahniuk)

17. Damaged

I loved going to Bridgewater State College. The campus was beautiful, the professors were great, attractive women were plentiful, and the three-story library had an endless supply of interesting books to read. The psychology section was my favorite. It had the complete works of Carl Jung and Sigmund Freud, two early psychoanalysts I greatly admired. I managed to read all of their books during my time at Bridgewater plus many, many others.

For the few years I spent at BSC, my days more-or-less followed the same pattern. I would get up, go to my classes, then spend most of the afternoon in the library. Sometimes I'd take a break from the library and go over to the music building for an hour or two. Even though I wasn't a music major, they'd let me get a key to one of the piano practice rooms if it wasn't in use. I'd play for a while and then go back to the library until the late afternoon. Then as soon as my friend Chris got home from work, I'd head over to his house for the evening.

Much like my days followed a similar pattern, so did my nights. I'd get to Chris's shortly after he got home from work and we'd go right to the packie. Every night we'd get the same thing: a thirty-rack of Bud Light, a pint of peppermint Schnapps, and a couple packs of Marlboro Reds. Then we'd go to Chris's house, fire up his wood stove, and put on the back-to-back reruns of The Simpsons that Fox played at the same time every night. By the first commercial break, the Schnapps would be gone. Then we'd slam beers, talk, laugh, and chain-smoke cigarettes for the rest of the night. Sometimes a bunch of our friends would show up. Other times it was just me and Chris. Either way, it didn't matter. We always had a good time.

    Chris had a little sister named Stephanie who was five years younger than me – almost to the day. Her birthday is just two days before mine. Sometimes she'd come hang out with us and I always liked having her around. Steph was cute, fun, and full of energy. When we first met, she was still in her mid-teens and I didn't see her as anything more than Chris's little sister. But by the time I graduated from Bridgewater, Steph was almost twenty – and I started seeing her as a lot more than just my friend's little sis.

    Late one night after breaking up with her boyfriend, Steph called my Nokia cell phone and asked me to come over. I did and we stayed up all night talking, kissing, and cuddling. Little did I know at the time, that night would be the start of the most tumultuous relationship of my life.

    Steph (or Stephanie II as I sometimes refer to her) and I started getting together every night after I got out of work. I'd finished college, received my bachelor's degree, and found a job working at a residential school for teens with special needs. Every night after work, I'd stop by the packie and grab enough alcohol for both of us to get absolutely shitfaced – and shitfaced we got, every night. Before long, we were living together.

    The first few months of our relationship were great. All we did was drink, laugh, and fuck. But then things changed. One night, I came home from work and Steph had invited two friends of hers to spend the night. They had nowhere to go so she said they could stay with us. Both of them were opioid addicts. One of them had a bunch of Percocet and gave me a few of them. That's all it took. It reminded me of how good it felt to take opioids. After that, I was off and running again.

    I started buying pills on the street and before long it evolved into full-blown opioid addiction. Steph had an equally-troubling drug problem, though she preferred uppers to downers. I was still seeing Dr. Karlin and he was still prescribing me The Magic Combo. However, I turned The Magic Combo into the Tragic Combo. Steph and I both had prescriptions for controlled substances and we both abused them. If I'd been smart, I would've stayed away from alcohol and opioids, and continued taking my meds as prescribed. But I didn't do that and the result was a downward spiral that almost killed me.

    After about a year of being with Steph, I'd had enough. As much as I loved her, I was starting to realize that we weren't good for each other. Our entire relationship at that point revolved around drugs and alcohol. Well, that and lies. But the lies always revolved around drugs and alcohol just like the rest of our relationship. I had been strongly considering packing up my stuff, breaking up with Steph, and moving out. Then one morning she came storming into our bedroom with some life-changing news.

    "Ellis," Steph said, kicking my leg. "Wake up. I've got something to tell you."

    "Tell me later," I replied, pulling the covers over my head, incredibly hungover from a long night of drinking with her brother.

    "I just went to the doctor," she said, kicking me again. "I thought you'd want to know: I'm pregnant."

"Greaaaaaat," I replied.

"You're un-fucking-believable," Steph said and stormed out of our bedroom, slamming the door on her way out.

"Whatever," I replied, rolled over, and fell back asleep for several more hours.

I'm not proud of my initial response, but that's how it happened. Steph gave me a lot of shit for the way I handled the news and I deserved it. When I woke up a few hours later, what she'd told me finally sunk in. I was going to be a father. But after pondering that thought for a moment, my attention was directed to a more-immediate concern. It was a new day and I was out of drugs. So I put Steph's pregnancy on the back burner and went out to go find my drug of choice.

For the first couple months of Steph's pregnancy, nothing really changed. We both continued to use drugs and drink all the time. I abandoned my plan to leave Steph and move out, since we were going to be having a kid together. My drug use continued to escalate to the point where I couldn't get out of bed without taking something. I was so desperate that there were mornings I'd send my pregnant girlfriend out to score some drugs for me. Even though the Behcet's seemed to be in remission, my health was deteriorating rapidly. I looked like a skeleton – and a very pale one at that. Everything from my mental health to my dental health was terrible. When I wasn't high, I had crippling anxiety and felt absolutely miserable. My mouth was filled with cavities from sucking down Mountain Dews and eating nothing but highly-processed, sugar-filled foods. I racked up thousands of dollars worth of debt, maxed out all my credit cards, and neglected my car's maintenance until it was no longer driveable.

I was a fucking mess – and I knew it. Even Steph, who was quite the train wreck herself, was worried about me. I recently had a conversation with my good friend Joe who knew me back then and we were reflecting on the past twenty years of our lives.

"I can't believe I just turned forty," I said to Joe in a lighthearted tone. "I never would've thought I'd live long enough to see my forties."

"I didn't think you'd live to see twenty-five," Joe replied with both sincerity and seriousness in his voice. "Honestly. None of us did. We were all worried about you, bro. Even Steph thought you were going to die and she was in rough shape herself."

Joe isn't the only one who's said something like that to me, but he's the most recent. Everyone who cared about me at the time was worried. The only thing I ever worried about, though, was getting more drugs. But then Steph came home with more news a couple months later that changed everything.

"It's a boy!" she said, storming into our bedroom, slamming the door behind her. Steph was a stormer and a slammer regardless of her mood.

"What?" I asked, taking my headphones off.

"It's a boy. We're having a little baby boy."

In an instant, it all became real. Like, *really* real. I wasn't having a kid. I wasn't having a baby. I was having *a boy*. All of a sudden the seriousness of it all set in. My girlfriend was pregnant with my son. My *drug-addicted* girlfriend was pregnant with my son. I looked over at the mirror and the cold, hard truth punched me right in the face. If Steph and I didn't make some serious changes to our lives – and make them fast – our son was going to have two drug-addicted losers as parents.

I went out drinking with a few guy friends that night to celebrate finding out Steph and I were having a boy. As always, I drank until I blacked out. And then for the second time that day, I was punched in the face. But this time it wasn't by the cold, hard truth. It was by a tightly clenched fist.   I was in the passenger seat of my friend's car with two others in the back seat. All of us had been out drinking and causing trouble all night long – all but one. Sitting behind the driver was Fred. He hadn't drank a drop of alcohol all night and didn't participate in any of our shenanigans. We were out driving around at two-in-the-morning and a cop pulled us over. Fred wasn't wearing his seat belt and the cop gave him a ticket. The rest of us, nothing. Though I don't remember any of this, I've been told that I laughed at Fred and started making fun of him as soon as the cop let us go. He apparently warned me that if I didn't stop running my mouth, he was going to hit me. Fred's a man of his word and I was a man who'd had way too much to drink. I didn't stop ragging on him. So he clocked me right in the mouth, chipping one of my already-brittle teeth.

By the time we got home, I was livid. I guess I'd been threatening to kick Fred's ass the whole ride back. Sure enough, as soon as we got out of the car, I started swinging at him. We ended up on the ground, our friends broke it up, and that was the end of that. Before that night, I never really liked Fred. But after the fight, we made up and my opinion of him changed. After we beat the shit out of each other that night, I started to respect and eventually even like Fred. To this day, I still consider him a friend. It's funny how that works out sometimes.

The next morning, I woke up with a hangover and a chipped tooth. But I also woke up with a new mindset. I guess getting punched in the face twice in one day – first with reality, then with a fist – was just what I needed.

I didn't want my son to have a fucking loser for a dad. I wanted my son to have a father he could look up to and be proud of. A positive role model instead of a negative one. I wanted to be able to take care of my son's needs, physical and emotional. Overall, I just wanted to be a good dad. And if I was going to do that, I knew I needed to make some serious changes to every aspect of my life.

> "The greatest discovery of all time is that a person can change his future by merely changing his attitude." - Oprah Winfrey

18. Negative To Positive

When Steph was about five months pregnant, we both wanted to get clean and knew that neither of us could do it on our own. So we each checked into a detox facility. I don't recall where she went, but I ended up at McLean Hospital in Belmont on their dual-diagnosis unit. McLean's is a world-famous psych hospital known for their cutting-edge research and highly credentialed staff. It's also where the book Girl Interrupted took place, which was later made into a film starring Winona Ryder. Good book, great movie.

Most of my time at McLean's was spent sleeping and eating. When I checked in, I only weighed one-hundred-and-thirty pounds – and I'm six-feet tall. They rapidly detoxed me off everything I'd been taking, prescription and otherwise. The whole time I was there, I had no energy and no motivation. My brain needed some time to get used to not having chemicals pumped into it every few hours. They quickly tapered me off everything until the only thing they were giving me was Suboxone. It's similar to methadone except it's harder to abuse and you don't swallow it – you let it dissolve under your tongue. The only other drug I was on at McLean's was nicotine. I don't remember how I got them in there, but I had a pack of Marlboros and a lighter with me. Even though it was clearly against the rules, I would sneak a cigarette in the bathroom when I showered in the morning and at night.

When I was at McLean's, I made a decision that would shape the rest of my life. Up until that point, I was incredibly negative. I always saw the bad in situations and in people. When I thought about the future, I assumed the worst would happen. When I thought about myself, I only saw my negative qualities. But can you blame me? When you've been living a life filled with pain and suffering for so long, it's almost impossible to *not* see the world in an overly negative way. But with the impending birth of my son, I was determined to change that.

Being at McLean's gave me a lot of time to clear my head, both literally and metaphorically. It gave me a chance to take a step away from myself and really examine the direction my life was going in. I knew if I didn't change the way I thought about the world, I'd never be able to change my life. Any outer change has to start from within. So I made the decision to change the way I talked to myself and the way I viewed the world altogether.

Instead of seeing the future as bleak, I'd see it as an endless ocean of opportunity. Instead of thinking of myself as a worthless loser, I'd think of myself as someone with immense potential. Instead of looking at the world as an endless source of pain and suffering, I'd look at is as a place filled with wonder, joy, and excitement. Instead of being destructive, I'd be creative. Instead of being consumptive, I'd be productive.

In other words, I decided to stop being so damn negative and start being more positive.

Of all the easier-said-than-done tasks I'd set my mind to over the years, this one would prove to be the most difficult. But it would also turn out to be by far the most rewarding. What started as simply identifying negative thoughts and replacing them with positive ones turned into a total-mind-and-body transformation.

Changing the way I thought about myself and the world was just the first part of my plan – a necessary part for what was to follow. When you think everything sucks and is always going to suck, it can be hard to find the motivation to put effort into bettering yourself. But once I started to see myself and my future in a more-positive light, I was able to slowly start making some changes to my *out*side world to match the changes I was making to my *in*side world.

The first positive change I made – the second, if you include getting clean – had an impact on *both* worlds and I got a jump on it before I'd even left McLean's. They had a small exercise room with some basic fitness equipment. I didn't have much energy while I was at McLean's, but I managed to go to the exercise room a few times. It's no secret that exercise can improve a lot of different things, from sleep to anxiety, energy levels to mood. So I made the decision to get myself a gym membership as soon as I got out of McLean's. And that's exactly what I did.

As soon as I finished my undergraduate degree in 2005, I got a job working at a residential program for teens with special needs. I'd been there for about two years when I checked myself into McLean's. They were cool enough to give me a few months off to rehabilitate myself. The head of my department was a recovering alcoholic and addict himself. He was happy to give me the time off to get my shit together. One of the benefits my employer offered was a fifty-percent-off membership to the local YMCA. After getting out of McLean's but before going back to work, I signed up at the Y and started going three times a week.

I really didn't know what I was doing when I first started working out. I'd made a few unsuccessful attempts to build some muscle in the past, but always gave up before seeing any real results. I knew about some basic lifts like the bench press and squats, but that was it. For the first several months I went to the YMCA, I'd do the few basic free-weight lifts I knew, use some machines for a while, and then get on the treadmill.

When I was first starting out, I could only walk on the treadmill for five minutes before feeling like I was going to drop dead. That's right: my cardio was so bad that I could only *walk* on the treadmill for five minutes at a time. Running was out of the question. Fifteen seconds of jogging was all my weak legs could tolerate before I had to quit. And my upper-body strength wasn't much better. I could barely bench press one-hundred pounds ten times. Your average twelve-year-old gymnast probably has more arm strength than I did. I was in pathetic shape for a twenty-six-year-old man, even for one with a chronic autoimmune disease.

But I kept going to the Y and I kept pushing myself. It wasn't easy. There were days I didn't want to go. There were times when I wanted to quit. But I kept going, pushing myself just a little harder each workout. Gradually, over time, I got stronger and my cardio improved. Before long, I could walk for fifteen minutes at a time and at a slight incline. All my lifts slowly went up and, after a few months, my strength progressed to the level of your average fourteen-year-old gymnast. I was making progress.

In the first nine-or-so months I went to the

gym, I put on about twenty pounds of muscle. I went from around a-hundred-and-thirty pounds to over one-fifty. But then I plateaued. My cardio continued to improve the more I pushed myself, but I wasn't getting any stronger and I wasn't building any more muscle. I also had a little bit of stubborn lower-belly fat that, no matter how much cardio I did, wouldn't go away. That's when I realized I needed to change something else: my diet.

I knew that protein was important for building muscle and had started trying to eat more of it when I first began exercising. But I didn't realize just how important it is or how much of it I needed to build more muscle. After doing a lot of research and talking to some people at the YMCA, I doubled my protein intake. In no time, my strength went up and I started building muscle again.

I also realized that, if I wanted to get rid of the last remnants of my skinny-fat body hanging around my lower belly, I needed to start eating less sugar – start *consuming* less sugar, I should say. A lot of the excess sugar responsible for my belly fat was coming not from what I ate, but from what I drank. The first thing to go was my beloved Mountain Dews. I stopped drinking soda everyday and only allowed myself a little bit on the weekends. That got rid of some of my belly fat. The next thing that had to go was the large French-vanilla coffee with extra cream and extra sugar from Dunkin' that I got every morning. Well, not the large French vanilla coffee. Just the extra cream and extra sugar.

I made a few attempts to switch to black coffee, but that didn't go so well. Every time I tried, it lasted for a few days until I went right back to loading it up with tons of cream and sugar. The switch from sweet and creamy to bitter and bland was too drastic for my taste buds. So I did the same thing with cream and sugar that I was doing with Suboxone: I gradually tapered my dose. I went from extra everything to extra cream and regular sugar. Once I got used to that, I started drinking my coffee with regular cream and regular sugar. After a few weeks of that, I switched to regular cream and two sugars. I kept going back and forth lowering my cream and sugar until, nine-months later, I was drinking my coffee black – and enjoying it.

    It wasn't long after my cream and sugar taper that I noticed most of my belly fat was gone. Cutting out all the sugary drinks I'd been regularly consuming for so long was enough to finally help me burn it off and keep it off. To this day, I still limit myself to one or two sodas a week. Other than the occasional soda and daily protein shakes, I generally try not to drink too many calories. Now I usually just drink unsweetened green tea, black coffee (French vanilla, of course), and water.

    Over time as I learned more and more about nutrition, I made more and more changes to my diet. I started eating more fruits and vegetables, less refined carbs and other processed foods, and more lean meats and dairy. Don't get me wrong: I still enjoyed myself, just like I do now. I've always had a sweet tooth: soda, pumpkin pie, and chocolate are among my favorite indulgences. But my all-time favorite? Malasadas. They are my ultimate weakness. If you don't know what a malasada is, it's Portuguese fried dough. Think regular fried dough, only sweeter and topped with regular sugar instead of powdered sugar. My grandmother was from San Miguel[1] and used to make them when I was a kid. For as long as I can remember, they've always been my favorite treat. If for some reason you ever need to bribe me with food, a malasada is your best bet.

Now and for the past several years, I've been following what I like to call the ninety-ten rule. Ninety percent of what I put into my body are healthy, clean foods: lean meats and dairy, fruits and veggies, and some whole grains. The other ten percent is whatever else I want: cookies, candy, cake, pie, soda and, of course, malasadas. I eat healthy most of the time, but still enjoy myself a bit, too. That is, after all, what life's all about – what my *new, positive* life was all about: being good to myself, having fun, and enjoying life... but doing so in a healthy, balanced way. It would still take me a few more years to really find true balance in my life, but it all started with the attitude change I made while at McLean's.

---

[1] San Miguel is part of the Azores, a group of islands off the coast of Portugal. It's also the island and Catholic saint I was named after.

"Since this is the age of science, not religion, psychiatrists are our rabbis, heroin is our pork, and the addict is the unclean person." - Thomas Szasz, MD

19. No Sex and No Drugs

A couple months after I got out of McLean's and Steph got out of whatever detox facility she'd been at, on a warm evening in May, our son was born. For the first time, I got to actually see and hold what – now a *who* – had been motivating me so powerfully to change my life. All the things I couldn't seem to do for myself, I *could* do for him. He finally gave me some direction after a lifetime of purposeless wandering. To this day, my son remains one of the biggest motivators in my life and I'm incredibly thankful that he came along when he did.

For the first six months after our son was born, Steph and I were a happy little family. We moved out of our small, shitty apartment and in with a friend and mentor of hers. By some miracle, our son seemed perfectly healthy in spite of Steph using throughout the first half of her pregnancy. We were both going to meetings[1] and doing everything we needed to do to stay clean. For those six months, things were good. It looked like everything might actually work out.

But then we began having problems. Steph started using again. I didn't. I was committed to my new healthy lifestyle. But she struggled and started going out a lot. I don't blame her – not anymore,

---

[1] Narcotics Anonymous (NA), Alcoholics Anonymous (AA), and my personal favorite, Smart Recovery.

anyway. I didn't even really blame her at the time. I knew how powerful the temptation could be. I fought it off daily and it certainly wasn't easy. But I did it which is all that matters.

Steph and I were on again, off again for a while. But there came a time when I had no choice but to give her an ultimatum. It was either me and our son or the drugs. One or the other, but not both. I knew deep down Steph wanted to do the right thing, but her actions made the decision for her. She couldn't help herself. So I had to do one of the hardest things I've ever done. After several years and more ups and downs than the stock market, I ended things with Steph. It broke my heart but I had no choice. It was the right thing to do for myself and, more importantly, for my son. That breakup left a bitter taste in my mouth that would linger for years. The only comfort I got was in knowing I did everything in my power to make things work. But it just wasn't enough.

After Steph and I broke up, I went through a period of remission – but not just from Behcet's disease. The Behcet's had already been in remission for a couple of years when her and I called it quits. I would also go into remission from drugs and dating.

To remit means to stop. When a disease goes into remission it means that, while still there, it stops being active. Behcet's disease often hits hard at first, then goes into remission for a while. For a lucky few it never comes back. For most like myself it will come back eventually. But at least I got to enjoy a few years without any symptoms.

There's really only one word to describe how I felt when Steph and I were finally done for good: devastated. It took me years to get over her and everything we went through together. Immediately following the breakup, I went out with one woman. It was a classic rebound situation. I needed to prove to myself that I was still desirable – and I did. But after that, I stayed away from women for the next five-or-so years.

When I left McLean's, I left with a single prescription: Suboxone. They took me off all the other meds I'd been on. Dr. Karlin, the psychiatrist I was so fond of, would continue to prescribe the Suboxone for the next couple months. But he had to refer me to another psychiatrist, Dr. Antonio Zheng, to prescribe the Suboxone because he was leaving CCBC, the place I saw him at. I really didn't want to stop seeing Dr. Karlin, but I had no choice.

I didn't like my new psychiatrist. Dr. Zheng had a wall full of degrees, diplomas, and board certifications, yet he didn't know the first thing about how to interact with his patients. And he treated me like a criminal. Every month when I went to go see him, I had to pee into a cup. It was embarrassing and I resented him for it. After all, it was doctors who got me hooked on opioids in the first place. To have one treat me like it was *my* fault was insulting.

My new psychiatrist continued prescribing me Suboxone and we gradually lowered the dosage over time. After seeing Dr. Zheng for a few months, I told him that I was having a lot of anxiety. He prescribed me Zoloft, a common antidepressant that is also approved to treat anxiety disorders. Though I'd never taken Zoloft, I'd been on several similar drugs[1] in the

---

[1] Other selective serotonin reuptake inhibitors (SSRIs) like Prozac (fluoxetine) and Celexa (citalopram). I'd also been on Effexor (venlafaxine), a selective norepinephrine reuptake inhibitor (SNRI).

past. None of them had ever done anything for my mood or anxiety and I told him that, but he insisted Zoloft was different. So after doing some research, I filled the prescription and decided to give it a try.

The next month, I reported back to Dr. Zheng. His assistant/wife had me pee into a cup, then brought me back to see her employer/husband. I told him that the Zoloft wasn't helping my anxiety. It didn't seem to be doing much of anything. Fortunately, I didn't experience any side effects like I had with the other SSRIs I'd been on in the past. The doctor wrote me a new Zoloft prescription, doubling the dosage. He said a higher one would help. I was skeptical but decided to try it. The doctor wrote me my Suboxone prescription and told me to come back in a month.

A month later, same thing. Pee into a cup, then back to the doctor's office. I told him that the Zoloft still wasn't doing anything. Dr. Zheng told *me* that I failed the drug test I'd taken the month before, testing positive for benzodiazepines. They're a class of anxiety-reducing drugs that include Xanax, Ativan, Valium, and Klonopin, among many others. I told the doctor that I hadn't taken anything other than what he was prescribing me, but he didn't believe me. He didn't even *pretend* to believe me. What he *did* do was write me another useless Zoloft prescription along with my Suboxone. He told me that sometimes it takes several months to work.

A month later, pee in a cup, then back to see the doc. Dr. Zheng told me that I tested positive for benzos again. And again, I told him I hadn't taken any. He still didn't believe me. The doctor told me that the tests don't lie. But I knew better. I'd heard countless stories of people testing positive for things they never took. They're called *false positives* and they happen all the time. Dr. Zheng told me that if I tested positive for benzos one more time, he would stop prescribing the Suboxone.

I was so pissed off when I left his office that I seriously considered getting my hands on some benzos and taking them. If I was going to be accused of something, I might as well be guilty of it. I also considered never going back to see him. But I had to for two reasons. One, I needed the Suboxone. Even though I'd been slowly lowering the dosage, I was still taking enough that I'd go through severe withdrawal if I suddenly stopped taking it. And two, I needed to prove that arrogant doctor wrong and wipe the condescending look off his smug face. So I went home, got on the computer, and did a ton of research, printing out my results.

The next month, I went back to see Dr. Zheng. After giving his wife my likely-to-fail urine sample, she brought me back to his office.

"Good morning, Mr. Michaels," the doctor said.

I didn't reply. I just walked up to his desk, slammed a stack of printed papers on it, and had a seat.

"What's this?" Dr. Zheng asked.

"Take a look and see for yourself," I said, leaning back in the chair and folding my arms. He pulled the stack of papers closer and started flipping through them. "It's proof that I haven't been taking any benzos. As you can see, Zoloft is known to cause false positives for benzodiazepines. And here are about twenty anecdotal reports of people on Zoloft testing positive for benzos when they didn't take any."

The doctor looked up at me briefly, then continued flipping through the papers.

"I've been telling you the truth," I continued. "I haven't taken any benzos since they took me off them at McLean's almost a year ago. I really wish you would've trusted me. Trust between a patient and his doctor is of the utmost importance."

"Well," Dr. Zheng said, looking up at me with a goofy grin, "I have to apologize, Mr. Michaels. I wasn't aware that Zoloft could cause false positives for benzodiazepines."

You'd think that with all those plaques on the wall, you would know something like that, I thought to myself.

"I guess we both learned something then," I replied.

What *I'd* learned was that I couldn't trust Dr. Zheng. I wasn't lying when I'd said that trust between a doctor and his patient is incredibly important. He learned that I *could* be trusted. And I leaned that he *couldn't*.

I told the doctor I didn't want to keep taking the Zoloft. I also told him that I wanted to taper off Suboxone more aggressively. It made the process of getting off a little harder, but I wanted to stop seeing him as soon as possible.

After stopping the Zoloft, my drug tests started coming back negative again. Dr. Zheng apologized to me for a second time, but the damage had already been done. I tapered off the Suboxone quickly over the next few months and stopped seeing him.

For the next five years, I didn't take any prescription meds at all. The only drugs I consumed were caffeine, nicotine, and rarely but occasionally alcohol. And by the time those five years were over, I'd only be consuming one of the three. I was so discouraged by my experiences with the psychiatrist that I stopped seeing doctors altogether. The primary care physician I'd been seeing since I became an adult had passed away from brain cancer a year earlier. I had to find a new PCP for my employer, who I saw just once to get a form signed, but that was it. And with no Behcet's symptoms, I didn't see any reason to keep seeing a rheumatologist or any other specialists.

For five years straight, I managed to completely avoid the medical system. I have to say, it was incredibly liberating. Granted, I was depressed and anxious the whole time, but at least I was free from a corrupt system that puts profits over patients. During those five years, in spite of the depression and anxiety, I continued to make some positive changes to my life.

I also made some big mistakes.

"When you smoke the herb, it reveals you to yourself." - Bob Marley

20. The Dark Ages

When I was on Suboxone, I didn't realize just how much it had been helping my mood and anxiety. While I was on it, I felt decent enough. But once I came off Suboxone, the depression and anxiety I'd dealt with for much of my life came back in full force.

For years, every day was a struggle. Sure, I was in remission from Behcet's disease. But I wasn't in remission from anxiety and depression. Just getting out of bed often required what felt like a heroic amount of effort. And my anxiety made being around people almost painful. Aside from going to work everyday, I mostly stayed in to avoid having to be around anyone. My weekday schedule was always the same: get up at the last-possible minute, force myself to get ready for work, drive to work overcome with dread about everything that could (but in all likelihood, wouldn't) go wrong throughout the day, slog through the workday hating every second of it, then go home and play video games or sit in front of the television until it was time to go to bed. Like so many others out there, I was miserable every single day.

My weekends weren't much better. Anxiety and depression don't seem to know the difference between a weekday and the weekend. During a typical week, I would pick up my son on Friday and have him until Sunday. I really tried my best to be a good dad but, with no energy and constantly worrying about everything, it wasn't easy. He was still just a baby, so it wasn't very hard to hide how much I was struggling from him. But I couldn't hide it from myself no matter how hard I tried.

This went on for years. Suffer through the work week, struggle through the weekend, then do it all over again. In spite of myself, I still tried to maintain the positive attitude I'd set my mind to while at McLean's. I certainly wasn't always successful. But I kept trying to be less negative and more positive as much as possible. And I did my best to continue working on myself, even though I barely had any energy or motivation.

For a while, maybe a year or so, I stopped going to the gym. My employer stopped offering the sizable YMCA discount and I barely had the energy to get out of bed, let alone work out. But a new, reasonably priced, twenty-four-hour gym opened up not far from where I lived. After getting a membership there, I started working out again. I'd lost some of the progress I'd made at the Y, but quickly got my strength and endurance back to where they had been.

I also made some other positive changes to my life during those dark years. At the age of thirty, after twenty years of being a smoker, I finally gave up cigarettes for good. I'd made several failed attempts to quit in the past and they never lasted very long. Looking back, I think being depressed actually helped me to finally quit. My depression was at its worst around that time. I didn't have the motivation or energy to do much of anything. Even getting up and going outside to have a cigarette required more effort than I usually had to spare. So it wasn't hard for me to give up most of my twenty-or-so daily cigarettes. The only time it was really hard was in the car. I'd always smoke two cigarettes on the way to work and one or two on the way home. Those didn't require any more effort than reaching into my pocket and rolling down the window. But as hard as it was, I set my mind to it and stopped smoking altogether, even in the car.

    A couple of years later, I decided to stop drinking alcohol. After getting out of McLean's, I didn't drink at all for the first year or two. Then I only drank a few times a year when my friends managed to twist my arm enough to get me out of the house. It was during those dark years that my social anxiety was through the roof and alcohol made being around people not only tolerable, but enjoyable. The only problem was that I didn't have an off switch. Once I got started drinking, I couldn't stop myself.

    At the age of thirty-one, I got arrested for driving under the influence of alcohol (DUI) – for the second time. My first offense had been over a decade earlier when I was still with Stephanie number one. I wasn't even old enough to drink legally when I got that first DUI and they hit me with an underage-possession-of-alcohol charge, too.

    In Massachusetts, if your second DUI is more than ten years after your first, they treat it like a first offense. You go through the same first-offender class and have to jump through the same hoops to get your license back. The only difference is that they make you install a breathalyzer in your car when you do get it back.

    That thing was fucking awful. For starters, it was really expensive. You have to pay to have it installed in your car. Then you have to bring it in every month to get it calibrated, which they charge you an arm and a leg for. And when your two years are up, you have to pay even more to get it uninstalled. But the cost wasn't even the worst part.

Breathalyzers malfunction all the time, especially in cold weather. If the device senses alcohol or thinks that it's being tampered with, it locks your ignition so the car won't start. Every time you blow into the breathalyzer, it makes a record of it. And then when you bring it in to get calibrated, all the information is uploaded to the RMV[1] and the courthouse.

Late one night, I came out of the gym after a two-hour-long workout. It was a cold New England winter night, well-below freezing. I blew into the breathalyzer and it gave a false positive result. The only thing I'd been drinking that night was water and lots of it. In fact, by that time, I hadn't had a drop of alcohol in almost a year. The obnoxious buzzing sound the breathalyzer made after I blew into it made my heart rate double instantly. With shaky hands – half from anxiety, half from the cold – I blew into it again. This time, the device thought I was tampering with it and locked me out of my car for thirty minutes. Fortunately I was outside my twenty-four-hour gym. But if I had been in the middle of nowhere and it prevented me from starting my car, I could've gotten frostbite or worse. There have actually been cases of people dying as the result of malfunctioning breathalyzers in sub-zero climates.

I hated having that thing installed in my car – especially after I'd already quit drinking. It wasn't the second DUI that made me decide to quit drinking, though. You'd think that would've been enough to make me realize I should stop, but it wasn't. I decided to quit drinking almost three-years after that second

---

[1] Registry of Motor Vehicles in Massachusetts.

DUI on my favorite holiday, the Fourth of July.

Every year there is a big fair and fireworks display on the Fourth of July one town over from where I grew up. It became a tradition for me and several friends to always go together. On that particular year, I ran into Steph, my son's mother. We ended up getting drunk and spending the night together. It brought back all the feelings I once had for her that I'd worked so hard to get over. The next day, I felt horrible. Part of it was the raging hangover from drinking way too much alcohol. But it was mostly regret from spending the night with Steph. I needed to make sure something like that never happened again. And the only way that I could guarantee it wouldn't was by quitting alcohol entirely.

In addition to *quitting* something negative (alcohol), it was around that time that I also *started* doing something positive. I know not everybody will think it's positive, but it's turned out to be very positive *for me*. At my job, I confiscated a small bag of weed from one of the young men I worked with. I stuck it in my pocket and forgot about it until I got home that night. I thought about flushing the weed down the toilet, which is what I usually would've done. But for some reason, I stashed it away in a drawer my bedroom.

When I was a teenager, I liked to smoke weed. But once I got into my early twenties, its effects stopped being pleasurable. Every time I smoked, it just gave me anxiety. Naturally, I stopped. There were a few times later on in my twenties when I tried it again, always while drinking. And every time, it just made me nervous and paranoid. So every time, I'd anxiously wait for the effects to wear off and I wouldn't touch it again for another couple of years.

A few weeks after confiscating the little bag of weed and stashing it in my room, I had the week from hell. I don't remember the details now, just that it was much worse than usual. When I got home from work at the end of that week, I remembered the stashed bag of weed. I don't know what possessed me to try it that night, but I'm glad I did. I only took two little puffs. Over the course of the next few minutes, all the worries of the week gently washed away. It put me in a good mood for the rest of the night and I slept like a baby.

Weed once again did for me what it had as a teenager. The timing couldn't have been better. Since I'd given up hard drugs years earlier, alcohol was the only thing I had to help me relax. When I decided to give that up, I had nothing. Weed was a much-healthier alternative to alcohol for me. Not only did it help me to relax, weed was great at treating the insomnia I'd dealt with off and on my entire life. It also helped to boost my appetite, which was a good thing. I'd never had a big appetite and cannabis helped me to get some extra calories – most importantly some extra protein – into my diet.

At first, I only took a couple puffs one-or-two nights a week before bed. But over time I started smoking more. It was always at the end of the day when I was in for the night and didn't have to drive anywhere. With two DUIs under my belt, I've made sure to never, ever, under any circumstances drive while high. To this day, seven-years later, I can honestly say I've never gotten behind the wheel after smoking. Nor have I *been* behind the wheel *while* smoking, which I know a lot of people enjoy. But to me, it's just not worth it. There was a young guy in my DUI class who hadn't been drinking at all the night of his arrest. But the cop who pulled him over smelled weed and, even though he didn't have any on him, charged him with DUI. The last thing I want is for that to happen to me.

Smoking weed helped both my anxiety and depression. Even though I only used it at night, it helped me to get through the day knowing I had something to help me relax after work. The appetite boost from the weed also helped me to start building some more muscle – but not at first.

In the first couple of months after I started smoking weed, I got the munchies *bad*. I'd stop at a convenience store after work every night and buy cookies, cupcakes, sodas, and other junk food. In the store, I told myself I was buying enough food to last at least a few nights. But once I got stoned, by the end of the night, it would all be gone.

Fortunately, it didn't take me long to get the junk-food devouring out of my system. After just a couple months of pigging out nightly, I noticed that the lower-belly fat I'd worked so hard to get rid of was making a rapid return. My desire to wolf down tons of food after smoking didn't change, but what I put into my body did.

I stopped buying so much junk food and started stocking up on protein-packed foods. Instead of pigging out on junk, I'd pig out on baked chicken breast, grilled salmon, leafy greens, and other healthy foods. Within a couple of months, my belly fat was shrinking and my arms, chest, back, and leg muscles were growing.

Over the next couple years, I put on another fifteen-or-so pounds of solid muscle. I was slowly starting to feel better. My depression and anxiety were still there, but they were gradually improving. I was starting to have a little more energy. Things were finally starting to get better. And that's when the Behcet's decided to come out of remission so it could start fucking my life up all over again.

"Next to love, balance is the most important thing." - John Wooden

21. Labyrinth

It was the spring of 2015. I'd switched to an overnight position at my work about six-months earlier, managing an all-boys dorm at a residential school. I'll tell you more about why I switched to overnights a little later in the book. One night I had a woman named Charlotte working with me. She'd only been there for a short time and I didn't know her very well. But Charlotte seemed nice and we got along fine. We were about halfway through our ten-hour shift. All the students were sound asleep and had been for hours. I was on my laptop and Charlotte was on hers. It had been a perfectly normal night until I got up to use the bathroom around 3AM.

Whoa! I thought as I stood up. *What the fuck?*

I couldn't stand up straight. My body felt like it was about to topple over the second I got to my feet. I took a step toward the bathroom and had to immediately brace myself against the wall. When I reached for the wall, I almost missed it. In addition to being off balance, the room was slowly spinning.

This is not good. What the hell is wrong with me? And what's that sound?

I noticed a high-pitched ringing coming from my left ear. It would've been hard not to notice. The ringing was loud. I took another step toward the bathroom. And another and another, the whole time using the wall for support. The trip from that chair to the bathroom was one I'd made a thousand times before. It couldn't have been more than ten paces. But that night it felt like a hundred. I glanced at Charlotte as I rounded the hallway corner and she didn't seem to notice me clinging to the walls, desperately trying to stay upright on my way to the bathroom. I finally made it, shut the door, and plopped down on the toilet.

Something's definitely not right. When I'm seated, I seem to be fine. But when I'm standing, my body feels like it's going to topple over. There's no way the ringing in my left ear is just a coincidence. There must be something wrong with my inner ear. I remember from my EMT days that inner ear injuries can cause severe balance problems. But this is just crazy. It came out of nowhere. I was absolutely fine when I got up to do bed checks less than an hour ago. Now I can barely stand up without falling over. What the fuck?

After peeing sitting down, I stayed seated on the toilet for another minute to collect myself. I was quite shaken up. There was no explanation for what was happening – or was there?

Oh, no, I thought as it hit me like a ton of bricks. *No, no, no. I haven't had any Behcet's symptoms in years. Please don't be the disease coming out of remission. Please be something else. An ear infection. Brain cancer. Anything but Behcet's.*

At the time I couldn't have know for sure. But I do now. There's no doubt in my mind that it was, in fact, the Behcet's.

I slowly worked my way down the hall and back to my seat in the living room. This time, Charlotte *did* notice that something was wrong.

"Is everything alright?" she asked.

"I'm just feeling a little dizzy is all. It's probably nothing to worry about."

"Okay. Well, if there's anything I can do,"

Charlotte offered.

"There might be, actually. I might ask you to transition the students to class in the morning if you don't mind. Assuming I'm still feeling dizzy."

"Yeah, sure. No problem."

The dizziness and ear ringing didn't improve before morning. I did end up asking Charlotte to bring the students to class. It wouldn't have looked very good, me stumbling my was across the campus and back.

As soon as I got out of work, I called my primary care physician. First of all, after years of not going to any doctors, I called to see if he was even still my PCP. And second, to make an appointment. Fortunately, he was still my doctor and his secretary managed to squeeze me in that day.

My old PCP, the one who'd passed away years earlier, had his own private practice in an small, old, two-story, run-down medical building. He had one receptionist and one nurse – both older women. All of his records were kept the old-fashion way: with pen and paper. And he was a lifelong United States resident who had been practicing medicine since long before I was born.

My new PCP couldn't have been more different. He worked in a massive, modern, four-story, state-of-the-art medical building. There were several receptionists and several nurses, all in their twenties and thirties. The receptionist who checked me in and out was drop-dead gorgeous and looked just like Kathleen Robertson[1] in her early twenties. Everything was done electronically. And my doctor

---

[1] If you don't know who Kathleen Robertson is, that's fine. Just know that – especially in her early twenties – she was fucking gorgeous.

was an Indian-born physician who's younger than me.

"Mr. Michaels," Dr. Banerjee said with his thick-but-easy-to-understand Indian accent. "Long time no see. It says you're having difficulty standing and are experiencing ringing in your ears. Is that correct?"

"That's right," I answered. "I think it might be related to Behcet's disease. Last night, out of nowhere, when I tried to stand up..."

Dr. Banerjee got up, walked around the exam table I was sitting on, grabbed a otoscope[2] from the wall, and began looking in my ear as I explained what'd happened. I'm pretty sure he stopped listening to me the second he stood up. I remember learning in college that doctors, on average, listen to their patients for only eleven seconds before either interrupting them or tuning them out to begin their own internal diagnostic monologue.[3]

"I think this is a simple case of labyrinthitis," Dr. Banerjee concluded after a quick peek into my ear. "Inflammation of the inner ear. It's not all that uncommon. It explains the vertigo, the tinnitus – everything."

"What's causing it?" I asked. "Will it go away?"

"It should go away within a few days. A couple weeks at most. Labyrinthitis is usually caused by a viral infection or by bacteria."

"What about Behcet's disease? Can that cause

---

[2] An otoscope (or auriscope) is the thing doctors use to gaze deep into your soul... Your ear, I mean – deep into your ear.

[3] Ospina, N., Phillips, K., Rodriguez-Gutierrez, R. Castaneda-Guarderas, A., et al. (2018). Eliciting the patient's agenda – secondary analysis of recorded clinical encounters. *Journal of General Internal Medicine*, 34:36-40.

labyrinthitis?"

I now know that it most certainly can.[4]

"There's no reason to think this is being caused by Behcet's. I'm going to prescribe meclizine, an antihistamine used to treat motion sickness. The medication should help with the vertigo. If it gets worse or hasn't resolved within about a week, come back and see me."

The medication *didn't* help with the vertigo. However, the dizziness and balance problems did get better over the next few days, eventually going away. What didn't go away was the tinnitus: the ringing in my left ear. It got better but didn't go away – and it still hasn't five-years later.

I've noticed when my insomnia kicks up and I haven't slept well for a couple of nights, the tinnitus gets worse. That's not terribly surprising, though. When I haven't been sleeping well, just about everything gets worse: my joints hurt more, my brain is foggier, I'm more anxious, and I just feel shittier overall. When my insomnia is particularly bad, the ringing in my left ear is loud *and* annoying. It starts, then stops. Starts again, stops again. It almost sounds like Morse code.

Beeeeeep. Beep. Beep. Beeeeeeeeep. Beeeeeep. Beep. Beeeeeeeeeeep.

Wicked annoying.

I now experience tinnitus in *both* of my ears. Fortunately, it's not constant and is usually mild. Most of the time it's barely noticeable, if at all. However, it usually *is* noticeable at night when the world falls silent. The only way I can get to sleep is

---

[4] Hain, T. (2020, Oct. 25). Autoimmune inner ear disease (AIED). Retrieved November 1, 2020 from https://www.dizziness-and-balance.com/disorders/autoimmune/aied.html

by having fan, air conditioner, or some other source of white noise in the background to drown out the ringing in my ears.

The onset of the tinnitus in my right ear didn't come on suddenly like the left, nor has it caused me any problems with my balance. And it's much milder. While I'm now sure the labyrinthitis in my left ear was the Behcet's saying hi for the first time in years, I can't be sure what's caused the ringing in my right. Could it be Behcet's related? Absolutely. But it could also be the result of what my parents warned me about all throughout high school.

"If you keep listening to your headphones that loud," my mother would said, "you're going to have hearing problems later in life."

"I can't help it if I like loud music," I'd reply.

Is at least some of the ringing in my ears due to listening to my Walkman with the volume always on ten and all the loud, live music I've enjoyed over the years? It's certainly possible. But there's no doubt in my mind the labyrinthitis in my left ear was the work of Behcet's. How can I be so sure? Because of what happened just a couple weeks later.

"My rhymes are like shot clocks, interstate cops and blood clots, my point is your flow gets stopped." - Talib Kweli

22. Not Again

Mild-to-moderate stiffness and soreness in both my back and left leg were an everyday thing ever since those first clots in my late teens. But in the early summer of 2015, just a couple weeks after the labyrinthitis in my left ear, I started having some soreness and stiffness in my right leg. I didn't think anything of it at first. Mystery pain was just something that happened and it usually went away on its own. This time it didn't. What it *did* do was get much worse – and fast.

Over the course of a couple days, my right leg started getting a little stiff and sore. This was something that happened to my legs, arms, and other parts of my body from time to time, but it almost always resolved on its own. There was no swelling or serious pain, so I had no reason to think that this time was any different. I couldn't have been more wrong. It was very different. A series of massive blood clots were forming all the way down my leg.

When I woke up one morning – a Saturday morning, of course – my leg had gotten a lot worse overnight. Now it was a bit swollen and I could only bend it about halfway. I should've gone to the emergency room that morning, but I didn't.

I'm sure it's nothing to worry about, I told myself. *If it doesn't start getting better by Monday, I'll make an appointment with my primary care physician. And if it gets worse before Monday, maybe I'll go to the ER.*

I spent all day Saturday limping around, popping ibuprofen and acetaminophen to take the edge off the pain. That's my go-to, non-opioid, painkilling combo: eight-hundred milligrams of ibuprofen and five-hundred-to-a-thousand milligrams of acetaminophen. It works great for all types of pain: headaches, dental pain, joint and muscle pain – but apparently not for multiple-deep-vein-thromboses (DVT) pain. The only thing that took the edge off was weed. I'm not sure if it helped the pain directly, but it definitely helped to take my mind off it.

When I woke up the next morning, my leg wasn't any better. In reality, it was actually a little worse. But I told myself what I needed to hear to stay home and not go to the ER, a place to be avoided at (almost) all costs.

Well, I thought to myself, *my leg definitely didn't get any better overnight. But I don't think it's gotten too much worse. I mean, yeah, it hurts more than it did yesterday. But I haven't taken anything for the pain yet today. And is it just me or is it a little more swollen than it was yesterday? Nah, it's not. When I compare it to my other leg, I can see that the difference is the same as it was yesterday. I don't need to go to the ER today. Maybe I'll make an appointment with my doctor tomorrow morning if it's not starting to get better.*

If I *probably* should've gone to the ER on Saturday, I *definitely* should've gone Sunday. But I did what so many of us do so well: I talked myself out of doing what I should've done out of fear. I was afraid I'd hear what was quickly becoming impossible to ignore: that after years of remission, the Behcet's was back and in full force. I'd had so many strange symptoms come and go on their own over the years that it was easy to tell myself this time was no different. I kept telling myself that my leg would get better on its own. And like a fool, I listened.

Monday morning finally came along. Not only had my leg not gotten any better, it was still getting worse. It was now as stiff as a board and even walking up a single flight of stairs was a challenge. I called my PCP's office and he was able to see me that day.

When I walked into the exam room, there was no doubt in my mind about the cause of my symptoms. I knew that blood clots were to blame for my painful, swollen leg. It felt just like the clots I'd had almost twenty-years earlier. I knew that they were the result of swollen blood vessels, courtesy of Behcet's disease. And now there was no doubt in my mind that the labyrinthitis I'd experienced a couple weeks earlier was also related to my diagnosis. The timing of what I knew to be clots confirmed what I'd already strongly suspected.

Going to my primary for the labyrinthitis a couple weeks earlier was the first time I'd stepped foot into a doctor's office in over five years. Even though I considered myself a veteran patient, I was out of practice. I'd forgotten that there were protocols to follow and boxes to check off. I just wanted the doc to give me what I knew I needed and send me on my way.

"What brings you here today, Mr. Michaels?" Dr. Banerjee asked.

"I'm experiencing thrombophlebitis in my right leg from Behcet's disease," I explained. "I need you to put me on a corticosteroid to reduce the the inflammation and a blood thinner to break up the clot."

"Well, hold on," he said. "First, we need to confirm that it's actually a clot."

"It is," I replied. "I'm sure of it. This isn't the first time this has happened. This looks and feels exactly like the last time I had clots."

"It certainly *looks* like it *could* be a clot," the doctor said. "But clots are rare for guys your age."

"They're rare for eighteen-year-old boys, too, but I got them then. Did I mention I have Behcet's disease?"

"Yes, but we need to confirm that it's actually a clot and not something else. I'll have my assistant call over to radiology at Morton Hospital and have them get you in for an ultrasound right away."

"You can't just give me some heparin and prednisone so I can go home?" I asked.

"I'm sorry, Ellis. Go to Morton. I'll make sure they get you in quickly."

They did get me in pretty quickly. As soon as the sonographer started smearing the gooey gel all over my leg, the smell instantly brought me back twenty years to my first ultrasound. I remembered the smell, the slimy feeling, and the anxiety of doing whatever I could to not get an erection. This time, that wasn't a concern. Don't get me wrong: the technician was very cool and somewhat attractive, but I was no longer a teenage boy overflowing with hormones. She methodically ran the ultrasound probe up and down my right leg. I could tell by the look on her face that the test was confirming what I already knew to be true.

After finishing with my right leg, she did my lower abdomen and around my crotch. Not only was I happy that her hand didn't brush up against my junk, I was also happy knowing the ultrasound was just about over – or so I'd thought. But then the technician started smearing gel all over my left leg.

"What are you doing?" I asked. "The problem is with my right leg."

"I know, sweetie," she replied. "But I have to do both."

"Why? I don't see why that's necessary."

"It's so the radiologist can compare the two legs," she explained. "Don't worry. It won't take long."

"Alright. If you must."

I shut my eyes, letting my mind wander a bit. The sonographer started running the probe down my left leg. It actually felt kind of nice. My right leg was in pain and it hurt when she pressed down in certain spots. But when she started doing my left, it almost felt like a massage – a weird, gooey massage. It helped me relax a little bit. But when I opened my eyes and saw the look on the ultrasound technician's face, I knew something was wrong. It was the same look she'd made while scanning my right.

"What is it?" I asked, picking my head up slightly. "What's wrong?"

"I'm really not supposed to say anything," she replied. "The doctor will discuss the results with you after I'm done."

"Come on. Please. Tell me *something*."

"I could get into a lot of trouble."

"Would you at least turn the monitor a little bit more so I can see it, too?" I asked.

"I'm really not supposed to," she replied and paused for a second. "But you've been really nice to me."

It's true. I had. Even though I was in pain and anxious as hell, I tried to be nice to her and everyone else I had to deal with that day. I always try to be friendly and treat everyone I meet with kindness and respect unless they give me a *really* good reason not to. Almost always, I get kindness and respect right back in return. And even though it's not the reason why I try to be nice to everyone, it often makes people a lot more likely to help me out when I need it most. The sonographer turned the monitor slightly and continued dragging the probe down my leg.

"I'm not a radiologist," I said as I looked at the monitor, "but it looks like I've got clots in my left leg, too."

She nodded, slightly.

"You can turn the monitor back around," I said, displaying as much of a smile as I could. "Thank you."

"You're welcome," the woman replied and smiled back. Like mine, hers wasn't quite a full smile. "And again, please don't say anything."

"Say anything about what?" I asked.

She smiled back. This time, fully.

Not only did I have a series of clots and severe inflammation in the deep veins of my right leg, I also had clots and inflammation in my left. My right leg was worse, for sure. But I was surprised to find out I had clots in my left as well since that leg didn't look or feel any differently than usual.

The ultrasound technician finished the scan and I thanked her one last time. She left the room to go find the radiologist, leaving me alone with my thoughts. I always knew that the Behcet's could come out of remission at any time. But some people with the disease get hit hard for a few years and then go into remission for the rest of their lives. For years, I'd hoped I was one of those people. As I laid alone in the exam room with my eyes shut, I now knew for a fact that I wasn't.

The radiologist came in and told me what I already knew: that I had massive clots running down both legs. I feigned surprise when he told me about the left leg. I'd only mentioned the swelling, stiffness, and pain in the right on the stack of paperwork I'd filled out. I didn't want him to suspect the ultrasound technician told me anything – and he didn't. The radiologist then said that he'd spoken to my PCP who wanted me to be admitted to the hospital so I could start treatment right away. It was nearing five-o-clock and my PCP's building would be closing before I could get back there. Reluctantly, I agreed to check myself into the same hospital for the same reason I was admitted almost twenty years earlier.

"Poisons and medicine are oftentimes the same substance given with different intents." - Peter Mere Latham

23. Doctor, Doctor

The cool ultrasound technician who'd let me sneak a peek at her monitor brought me a wheelchair and pushed me from radiology to the emergency room at Morton Hospital. Even though her and I both made attempts to get all the ultrasound goo off me, I could still feel a little bit in my crotch when I slowly lowered myself into the wheelchair. And the smell lingered long after she left me in the ER. Every time I used the bathroom that night, long after it'd all dried up, I'd get a whiff of the pungent gel.

She wheeled me through the ER waiting room, past maybe a dozen people who looked about as happy to be there as I was. I could tell by their body language some of them had been waiting for a long time. They eyed me with disdain as I cruised right past them through the double doors into the ER. While they just showed up at the restaurant hoping to get a table, I had a reservation. I don't know if it was my primary care physician or the radiologist, but one of them contacted the ER and let them know I was coming. They already had a room waiting for me when I arrived. But that room basically turned out to be a one-person waiting room with a bed.

I sat alone in that room for a couple of hours, waiting to actually be admitted to the hospital. The ER doctor gave me some IV Dilaudid[1] to keep me

---

[1] Dilaudid (hydromorphone) is a powerful opioid used for moderate-to-severe pain.

comfortable. While it didn't completely kill the pain in my leg, it did make it a little more tolerable. Eventually, they wheeled me up to my second-floor accommodations.

The first time I was admitted to Morton with blood clots, I was there for almost a week. I really didn't want to spend another week there and was relieved when the attending physician told me they'd likely only keep me overnight. When I was admitted as a teen, they didn't know what was wrong with me. This time they did. The attending got me started on heparin injections right away. He gave me a quick lesson in subcutaneous (under the skin) self-injections and watched me do the first one. After using an alcohol pad to wipe my belly, I pinched my skin and pushed the needle in. I barely felt a thing. I'm glad I don't have a fear of needles because I'd have to jab myself in the belly a few times a day for the next week.

I really liked the overnight doctor who came in a few hours later. She was great. Not only was she really cool, smart, fun to talk to, and quite attractive – she was happy to give me whatever I wanted to keep me comfy.

"How's the Percocet working out for you?" she asked.

"Surprisingly, it's actually working a little better than the Dilaudid they gave me when I was waiting in the ER," I replied. "That barely took the edge off. But I didn't want to ask for more cause I didn't want to come across as a drug seeker. I was on opioids for over a decade so, even though I haven't taken them in a long time, I guess I may still have some sort of tolerance to them."

"You want me to increase the dose of the

Percocet?" she asked.

"That would be great, if it's no trouble," I replied.

"No trouble at all. You're due for your next dose soon. I'll have the nurse bring you two instead of just one."

"Awesome," I said and smiled. "Thank you."

"You're very welcome," the doctor replied and smiled back. "How about sleep? You want me to have the nurse bring you an Ambien?"

"Because I like you," I answered with a half-smirk, "I'm going to have to say no to the Ambien. I don't want to cause you any trouble."

"Trouble?" she asked with one raised eyebrow.

"Double trouble, actually," I replied, trying to keep my half-smirk from turning into a full-smirk. "If I took an Ambien, you'll likely have two issues to deal with. One, you'll have to deal with me limping up and down the hall looking for something to eat half the night. And two," I said now with three-quarters-of-a-smirk, not-so-subtly eyeing the doctor up and down, "you'll have to deal with me relentlessly trying to flirt with you until the sun comes up."

She laughed and said, "Yeah, Ambien can have some strange side effects. You've been on it before, I take it?"

"I have, yes. Sometimes it works great. I take it, lay down, and gently drift off to sleep. Other times I take it and get either super hungry or super horny – or both. So it's probably best if we skip the Ambien – for your sake. I'll take fifty milligrams of Seroquel, though, if that's cool."

"Sure," she replied, flashing another smile.

"That's fine. I'll have the nurse bring that and your Percocet in shortly. Hopefully you'll sleep through the night and be out of here tomorrow."

"Let's hope so," I replied with a smile. "Thanks again."

Shortly after the doctor left the room, a nurse came in with the Percocet and Seroquel. They worked like a charm. The Percocet helped to dull the pain in my leg enough that, if I laid in the right position, it was barely noticeable. And the Seroquel, something I'd been on for insomnia years earlier, helped to quiet my mind enough that I gradually drifted off to sleep.

The next morning I was happy to find out the treatment had started working. The doctors were, too. My leg was still far from normal, but it was no longer as stiff as a board. I could at least bend it a few degrees, something I couldn't do the night before. They said I could be discharged that day which, of course, was music to my ears. I made a couple of phone calls to find someone to pick me up, got started on the unnecessarily large stack of discharge paperwork, and a couple hours later I was out of there.

The first thing I did when I got home from Morton Hospital was exactly the same thing that I did when I got home from Morton nearly twenty-years earlier. Well, maybe not *exactly* the same. When I was eighteen, the first thing I did was go outside to smoke a cigarette – a regular tobacco cigarette. This time, I also went outside and smoked a cigarette. But instead of tobacco, it was a marijuana cigarette. I rolled up a fat joint, used the crutches the hospital had given (sold) me to go outside, sparked it up, and got lost in thought.

As I sat there smoking and thinking, the

reality of my situation set in. I knew that my doctor-and-medication-free streak was over. After years of staying away from doctors, I had no choice but to start seeing them again.

I had a follow-up appointment with my PCP the day after I got out of the hospital to figure out where to go from there. We both agreed that I should schedule an appointment with my old rheumatologist since the Behcet's was clearly no longer in remission. The doctor wrote me another Percocet prescription for the pain. The hospital only gave me a couple of days worth and, though it was starting to feel a little better, my leg still hurt quite a bit. And he also wrote me a prescription for Coumadin, the same blood thinner I'd been on as a teen.

Being on Coumadin sucks for several reasons. First, there are a number of foods that can affect how the drug works. You have to be as consistent as possible with several foods, especially leafy greens and other foods high in vitamin K. Second, Coumadin makes you bruise easier and bleed more if you get a cut. So you have to avoid contact sports and be extra careful when using knives, scissors, and other sharp objects. And lastly, the thing that sucks the most, you have to get frequent blood work to make sure you're not taking too much or too little Coumadin. Take too little and your clots could worsen. Too much and a paper cut could become a life-threatening injury.

I called my old rheumatologist's office to make an appointment with him. They told me that his schedule was full for several months but could get me in sooner if I saw one of his partners. I agreed. A week-or-so later, I saw the-only-of-the-three rheumatologists in their practice I'd never met before: Dr. Schwartz. I didn't know him, but he knew me.

Apparently, the reputation I'd established as a teen was still well known there. Behcet's is rare even among rare diseases, especially in the US. I asked Dr. Schwartz how many patients they had with Behcet's disease and he told me that I was only one of three. And only two-of-the-three cases – mine being one of them – were definitely, without question, Behcet's. So between the rare diagnosis, the rebellious attitude, and the long dreadlocks I had as a teen, it's not hard to understand how they might remember me.

  I liked Dr. Schwartz. That was the only time I've seen him. After that, I went back to seeing my old rheumy, Dr. Sack. He popped into the exam room for a few seconds to say hi when I was there with Dr. Schwartz. It was nice to see Dr. Sack after not seeing him for over half a decade. He and Dr. Schwartz briefly discussed my treatment plan outside the exam room. Dr. Schwartz had suggested to me that I start taking azathioprine, an immunosuppressant, before Dr. Sack had come in. When Dr. Schwartz returned to the exam room, he told me that Dr. Sack agreed azathioprine was the way to go. I took the prescription and told him I'd have to do my own research before I'd start taking it. But if I looked into it and agreed it was the right play, I'd fill the azathioprine prescription and start taking it.

  I never put any drug, prescription or otherwise, into my body without first doing a ton of research. I've always been a science nerd and actually enjoy reading medical journals, clinical trials, and other scientific literature (I'm weird. I know). Twenty-years earlier, my educational resources were limited to a dated copy of the Physician's Desk Reference (PDR)[1], a medical encyclopedia, and in college the one-or-two scientific databases my school library had. Now with the internet, I have access to everything – literally everything. Not only can I access pretty much every medical journal on the planet, I can read about firsthand experiences from other patients.

Azathioprine has been around since the 1950s. A lot of research has been done on the drug, including lots of research into its effect on the symptoms of Behcet's disease. Unfortunately, much of that research has been conducted in non-English-speaking countries where Behcet's is much more common. I went so far as to pay to have a few studies translated into English: some from Turkish medical journals, one from an Iranian journal. Behcet's is much more prevalent in those countries than it is in the US. After properly educating myself on how azathioprine works, its effectiveness at treating Behcet's, and reading reports from hundreds of patients who have taken it, I decided to fill the prescription. Even though azathioprine can have some serious side effects including increased cancer risk, there's a lot of evidence that shows it can significantly reduce the symptoms of Behcet's. In particular, azathioprine seems to be especially effective at reducing the incidence of eye problems, something I really want to avoid.

Speaking of eyes, Dr. Schwartz also suggested I schedule and appointment with an ophthalmologist. I agreed it would be a good idea. As much as I hated having my eyes poked and prodded, it had been over a decade since my last eye-doctor appointment. I

---

[1] The PDR was a big, annually-updated book of all the FDA-approved drugs doctors prescribe. It was considered the go-to reference for drug information by prescribers.

wanted to make sure there wasn't any new inflammation in my eyes since the disease decided to come out to play again.

Within a month, I went from not seeing any doctors or taking any meds for over five years to being hospitalized, seeing three doctors, and taking several meds within only a couple of weeks. I wasn't thrilled about my situation, but the positive attitude I'd worked so hard to cultivate allowed me to not only accept it, but make the most of it. And that's exactly what I did.

"Do more than belong: participate. Do more than care: help. Do more than believe: practice. Do more than be fair: be kind. Do more than forgive: forget. Do more than dream: work." - William Arthur Ward

24. Write

About a year before the Behcet's came out of remission, I'd made yet another positive change to my life. Ever since I was a little kid, I'd always been an avid reader. My entire life, I always dreamed about being a writer. I absolutely loved the idea of earning a living with my writing. Though I'd been a columnist for my college newspaper and got a couple of short pieces published in my early twenties, I never pursued my dream. But in 2014, I finally decided that it was time to turn that dream into a reality.

I'd been working at the same place for ten years. Ever since finishing my undergraduate degree, I'd been working at a residential school for teens with special needs. My job title and responsibilities changed a couple times over those ten years, but I always worked during the day either on first-or-second shift. And while I sometimes had short periods of downtime during my workdays, they weren't long or consistent enough to accomplish much of anything. But if I switched to third shift, I'd have plenty of time to myself.

The residences where the students lived were staffed twenty-four hours a day. At night during third shift while the students were sleeping, overnight staff were free to spend their time however they'd like. Their only responsibility was to do periodic bed checks to make sure the students were safely asleep in bed. The overnight shift was ten hours long. And of those ten hours, only two-to-three of them were spent actually working. The rest of the time while the students slept was yours to spend however you'd like.

    I decided to switch from working during the day to working overnights so I'd have time to get started on my new career – my dream career – as a writer. I'd always been a night owl and was up half the night anyway. So I sat down with the program director, told him I wanted to switch shifts and, a couple months later, I started working the graveyard shift. I had to take a slight pay cut, but it was very slight because I agreed to take an overnight management position. I'd still have plenty of time to myself, but I had more responsibilities than regular overnight staff. My job was to manage an all-male residence of seven students and one-or-two staff working under me.

    The overnight shift started at ten-thirty at night and got over between eight and eight-thirty in the morning. From about midnight to six was my writing time. Every night, after making sure the students were settled in for the night, I'd break out my laptop and get to work. I also spent a lot of time working on my new career at home, especially on the weekends. This wasn't just some little hobby I was taking up. I wanted to become a professional writer who was able to support himself with his writing. So I really gave it my all.

    When I was hospitalized with the clots in the late spring/early summer of 2015, I had no choice but to take a few months off from my overnight position. Had I gone to the hospital and started on blood thinners when my leg first started swelling up, I probably would've only had to be out for a week or two. But since I let my leg get really bad before starting treatment, it took a long time to get better.

At first, being stuck at home in bed bummed me out. I missed my friends at work and the gym. I missed being out in nature. And I just missed being mobile in general. But I didn't let it bum me out for long. I decided to do what I was starting to learn to do so well: turn a negative into a positive. Instead of sitting around feeling sorry for myself, I would use my time at home in bed to double down on my still-new writing career.

The first couple years of my new profession were mostly spent writing short pieces of non-fiction. I'd learned how to create websites and profit from them. When I got the clots in 2015, I was spending most of my writing time on a fitness website. But being stuck at home in bed made it hard to find the motivation to write about fitness. It made it hard to find the motivation to write about anything, really. But I summoned the positive attitude I'd worked so hard to craft over the years. Instead of seeing myself as a victim, instead of seeing things negatively, I'd look for the positive in my situation. And that positivity, I realized, came in the form of life's most-precious-yet-most-highly-undervalued asset: time.

Being out of work and not being able to exercise gave me a lot of free time, time I could use to start new projects and double down on old ones. But I didn't see it that way at first. I caught myself focusing on the negative: all the things I *couldn't* do. I couldn't exercise. I couldn't see my friends at work. I couldn't even go for a leisurely stroll around the neighborhood. By focusing only on the negative like the old me would've done, I quickly became saddened by my situation.

But then, after giving myself a couple of days

to feel sorry for myself, I pulled my head out of my ass. When something bad happens, I think it's okay to let yourself feel bad for a moment or two. But then you have to shake it off and keep moving forward, otherwise you risk getting trapped. Instead of focusing on the negative and all the things I *couldn't* do, I shifted my focus to the positive and what I *could* do. Without having to work or go anywhere, I had tons of free time. So I used that time to learn new skills and work on projects I hadn't had time for. Working on those projects and learning new skills gave my life meaning, something to get me out of bed in the morning. Okay, maybe not *literally* out of bed. I still had massive clots in both legs, after all. But they gave me something to wake up with enthusiasm for.

That's one of the secrets to living a happy life. You need to find meaning and purpose. You need a reason to wake up in the morning. Viktor Frankl in his book Man's Search For Meaning said that finding purpose in your life is the key to finding happiness. He was a doctor and a Nazi-concentration-camp survivor. Dr. Frankl noticed that some people in the camps, despite all their pain and suffering, were somehow able to maintain a positive attitude. All of those people, he observed, managed to find purpose in their suffering. They would spend their time trying to comfort others, sometimes even giving away their last piece of bread. Dr. Frankl found that the prisoners who survived the longest weren't the ones who were the fittest physically: they were the ones who maintained a positive attitude and found meaning in their miserable day-to-day lives. While I was bedridden with the clots, I used the writing projects I'd been working on as *my* purpose and it gave my life meaning. It helped me to stay positive in spite of everything I was going through.

Another thing I spent a lot of time on while stuck in bed was researching Behcet's disease. While in remission for all those years, I'd spent very little time thinking about the disease and even less learning about it. It was a classic case of ostrich syndrome: I stuck my head deep in the sand in the hope that the disease would just go away. Obviously, it didn't. Between the pain and swelling in my legs, all the doctor appointments, all the medications, all the blood work, and being stuck in bed, the fact that I had Behcet's was undeniable.

Instead of letting those constant reminders get me down, I used them as motivation to learn as much as I could about Behcet's disease. I wanted to know everything there was to know about this shitty illness. When I was younger, I'd read the few books about Behcet's that existed. But now with the internet, I had access to a lot more information. I familiarized myself with the websites of organizations like the American Behcet's Disease Association (ABDA) and Behcet's UK (formerly the Behcet's Syndrome Society). I combed through medical journals from around the world, reading about everything from new treatments to data about prognoses. And most importantly, I discovered a few Behcet's disease Facebook groups.

I was late to join the Facebook party. For years I resisted the idea of social media despite several friends trying to convince me to join. But when I started my writing career, I realized that learning to use social media was a necessity. Reluctantly, I created a Facebook account. It didn't take long for me to get hooked just like pretty much everyone else I knew. When the clots hit in 2015, I'd only been on Facebook for maybe a year. I was already a member of several fitness, nutrition, and guitar groups. While stuck in bed with the clots, I got the idea to search for Behcet's disease groups. I honestly wasn't expecting to find much. I thought maybe there'd be a small group with a handful of barely active members. But I was pleasantly surprised to find that there are several large Behcet's groups filled with activity.

I joined six different Behcet's groups on Facebook. Five of them currently have more than two-thousand members and one of them has close to five thousand. Since getting diagnosed, I felt like I was the only one on the planet with this lousy disease. Those Facebook groups not only made me feel less alone, they made me feel like I was part of a community. Our suffering bonded us all together in a way that couldn't possibly be understood by anyone without Behcet's. Not only have I learned a ton from those groups, I've made a lot of great friends over the past few years.

Having other people to talk to who have gone through and continue to go through what you have makes living with Behcet's suck a little bit less – a lot less, really. In some ways, it almost makes having the disease cool. It's like you're a part of this small club you have to earn your way into by going through the pain and agony of living with a body that won't stop attacking itself. No one else, no matter how honorable their intentions, can ever know what we know. Well-meaning parents, siblings, spouses, doctors, nurses, friends: they'll never truly understand what it's like to be us. Only other people who have Behcet's disease can know what it's like – and that bonds us all together.

"Sometimes pain was like a storm that came out of nowhere. The clearest summer could end in a downpour. Could end in lightening and thunder." - Benjamin Alire Saenz

25. Stomach Pain on the Fourth

As I may have mentioned, the Fourth of July is my favorite holiday. Fireworks trump parades, candy corn, turkey, and even presents. There's just something awesome about seeing a kickass fireworks display. Every year, ever since I was in my early twenties, a large group of friends and I get together every Fourth. Some of those friends, it's the only time I get to see them all year. Unfortunately, I didn't get to see any of them on the Fourth of July in 2015.

I was still out of work from the clots but my legs were feeling better. That day, I remember being anxious about going to the fireworks. I always parked at my friend Chris's house and so did everyone else. We'd all walk downtown together to watch the show. It's more-than-a-quarter-but-no-more-than-a-half-mile walk. For more than a month, the only walking I did was from my car to either a doctor's office, pharmacy, or lab for blood work, and then back to the car. And even then, sometimes it was a struggle limping my way through CVS to pick up my prescriptions. It's no accident they make you walk past all the yummy treats on your way to the pharmacy. And when you're limping along at only half your normal speed because you've got clots in your legs, it's almost impossible to resist the urge to grab a Snickers or a bag of Sour Patch Kids as you limp your way through the store.

All day long, I worried about having to walk from Chris's house to the fireworks and back.

What if I can't make it? What if my legs get really stiff and start to hurt so badly that I can't walk? Should I skip the fireworks this year? I know everyone will understand.

I really didn't want to miss the fireworks. And I didn't want to miss what might've been the only opportunity to see certain friends that year. Fred, the guy who'd punched me in the face nearly a decade earlier, was one of them. He'd been living in Pennsylvania and was coming up to join everyone for the fireworks. I would've loved to have seen him and all my other friends. But I really wasn't sure if I'd be able to make the walk from Chris's house to downtown and back. Gradually, I tried to ignore my anxiety and replace it with positive self talk, psyching myself up.

I'm going to go. I'll be fine. If my legs start hurting, I can just sit down for a few minutes. My friends will understand. I've never let this stupid disease stop me from doing what I want to do before. I'm not going to start now. Fuck it. I'm going. I'm definitely going.

And that was that. I decided I was going to the fireworks. I knew it would likely be a struggle. But I'd get through it and at the end of the day be glad I did.

As the afternoon turned into the evening and it got closer to the time I needed to get ready to go, my stomach started to hurt. It was mild and dull at first – certainly nothing to worry about. And I didn't. I just figured it was a little nausea from the azathioprine and Coumadin. Ever since starting them, I'd been having some nausea off and on. It usually wasn't very severe and always went away after a little while. But on the evening of the Fourth, the discomfort in my stomach didn't go away: it just lingered for hours.

The time came to get ready. I had a small snack hoping it would make my stomach feel better. It didn't. I took a quick shower, got dressed, and hopped in the car to make the fifteen-minute drive to Chris's house. And that's when the discomfort in my stomach turned into straight-up pain.

With every mile I drove, the pain got worse. Droplets of sweat began trickling from my forehead down the sides of my face. I loosened my seat belt to see if that would help. It didn't. I loosened my actual belt and undid the button on my shorts. That didn't make much of a difference either. The pain in my stomach continued to get worse, but I kept going. I got all the way to Chris's street until I couldn't take it anymore.

"Fuck!!!" I shouted out my car window. After taking a deep breath I continued talking to myself out loud, but in a calmer tone. "I can't do this. I need to get home. There's no way I'm going to be able to walk to the fireworks like this. I need to lay down. I tried. I really did. There's being courageous and then there's being foolish. I've got to get home. Fuck."

I was only thirty-seconds away from Chris's house when I turned around. For a moment, I felt like a failure. But my stomach was kind enough to take my mind off how disappointed I felt. What had started as mild, dull pain was now sharp and severe. My stomach felt like I'd swallowed a hummingbird with thumbtacks strapped to its wings.

And that's when I remembered the stomach pain I used to get as a child after having forgotten about it for nearly thirty years.

The feeling in my stomach was identical to the mystery pain I used to get as a little kid. It would start off dull. Then it'd get insanely painful out of nowhere and I'd curl up into a ball and cry. While the thought of pulling over, getting in the back seat, curling into a ball, and crying my eyes out like I would've as a child did have a certain appeal to it, I held it together and drove home. Well, I held it together as best I could.

"Fuuuuuuck!!!" I yelled every once in a while.

I remember reading somewhere that swearing actually makes pain easier to tolerate. It certainly seemed to that night. The whole ride home, in between outbursts of curse words, I thought about the stomach pain I used to get as a child. I couldn't believe I'd forgotten about it. If I'd told my doctors as a teen, maybe it would've helped them to make a diagnosis sooner. All of a sudden, it all clicked. The stomach pain I'd experienced as a child wasn't mystery pain: it was inflammation from the Behcet's. I already knew the disease had been active since at least my preteens. But now I realized it'd started even earlier than that. The satisfaction of solving a thirty-year-old mystery was almost distracting enough to take my mind off the pain in my stomach.

Almost.

"Fuuuuuuuuuuuuck!!!"

The fifteen-minute drive home felt like it took hours. Sharp, stabbing pain continued to torment my belly the whole ride, but I somehow made it home. After limping in the door hunched over and holding my stomach, I looked through the medicine cabinet for something that would help. I found a bottle of Pepto-Bismol, measured out a dose, and gulped the pink liquid down my throat. Then I laid down on the couch and curled up into a ball. No crying, though. Just curling. And maybe the occasional swear or two (or ten).

After maybe fifteen-or-twenty minutes, the pain started to get a little better. I took another swig of Pepto and laid back down. Fifteen-minutes later, it was starting to feel much better. I took one last dose of the thick, pink drink, put on the TV, and laid down again – this time on my back.

That stomach pain brought me right back to my childhood, lying in bed in the house I grew up in late at night, curled up, crying. I couldn't help but wonder if maybe the anxiety I'd been having all day brought it on or if it just happened out of nowhere. Ultimately, I came to the conclusion that they were unrelated. I'd had plenty of anxiety-filled days, many of them much worse than that Fourth of July. Yet none of them were ever accompanied by any stomach pain, especially not the intense pain I had that day.

The Pepto-Bismol dulled the pain enough that I was able relax and enjoy the rest of my night. I was disappointed I didn't get to see my friends, but I knew there'd always be next year. And I *did* join them the following year. When I woke up on the fifth, my stomach was completely back to normal.

After what I went through on the Fourth, I decided to start keeping a bottle of Pepto-Bismol in the backpack I brought with me everywhere I went. And it's a good thing I did. A few months later, my stomach started to hurt just as it had on the Fourth of July. It started out as dull, mild discomfort and then quickly started to turn into sharp, stabbing pain. Fortunately, I had the Pepto with me. I took a couple swigs before the pain got too severe and the Pepto-Bismol made it much better. That was about five-years ago and I haven't had any more severe stomach pain since. But to this day, I always carry a bottle of Pepto in my backpack just in case.

As much as it sucked going through what I did on the Fourth of July, I'm almost glad that I did – almost. If it wasn't for that day, I wouldn't have remembered the pain I used to get in my stomach as a kid. There are few things in life more satisfying than solving a puzzle, especially a thirty-year-old puzzle. I remember my five-year-old self lying in bed crying, looking up at the ceiling, and begging God for an answer:

"Why, God, why?" I asked, shaking one hand angrily at the ceiling, the other firmly grasping my aching stomach. "Why is this happening to me? Why are you doing this to me? Why would you put me through such agony? What did I do to deserve this torture?"

It took me thirty years to get an answer. Like they say: better late than never. But the answer didn't come from God himself. I'm still waiting to hear back from the bearded guy in the sky on that one – and every single other time I begged him for help. But now I had an answer. Now I knew. It wasn't some malevolent and sadistic god torturing a child for his own pleasure. It was the terrible autoimmune disease I couldn't have possibly known was lurking inside my body. I was too young to even spell *autoimmune*, let alone know what that term meant. But I do now. And as I learned from one of my favorite childhood cartoons that was on during the mystery pain years: knowing is half the battle.

"Grant me the serenity to accept the things I cannot change, the courage to change the things I can, and the wisdom to know the difference." - Reinhold Niebuhr

26. The Summer of Acceptance

The summer of 2015 was a major turning point in my life. I'd say that, in my adult life at least, it was second only to the spring of 2007 when my son was born. Like the months surrounding my son's birth, the months following the severe blood clots I got in 2015 were filled with inspiration, motivation, and reprioritization. Being out of work and stuck in bed all summer gave me plenty of time to think about what I really wanted in life. And the clots were a constant reminder to chase those dreams with everything I've got while I've still got it.

It wasn't until that summer that I finally, truly, one-hundred-percent accepted that I have, have always had, and will always have Behcet's disease. Don't get me wrong: I knew I had it. But I never *fully* accepted that I had it. I always tried to ignore it, to put it out of my mind in the hopes that it would just go away and never come back. When it *did* come back, I had no choice but to finally accept it. And I took things one step further. I didn't just *accept* that I had Behcet's disease: I *embraced* it.

Having others to talk to in Behcet's disease Facebook groups made a huge difference. I was no longer just some dude with a weird, fucked-up illness. I was one of *many* dudes and dudettes with the *same* weird, fucked-up illness. Behcet's was no longer something to be ashamed of and embarrassed by. It was something that would bond me with others from around the country and around the world. And that has made all the difference.

    I scheduled appointments with several specialists during the months I was home in bed. I'd already had my first rheumatology appointment with Dr. Schwartz, an associate of Dr. Sack, the rheumy I saw throughout my teens and early twenties. Next, I needed to make an appointment with an eye doctor to make sure everything was good with my precious peepers.

    I did a Google search for ophthalmologists in my area to see who the top-rated eye doctors were. Guess who was not only the closest but also the highest rated? The same on-call ophthalmologist who I had to drag away from his garden nearly twenty-years earlier. My initial reaction to seeing his name was less than positive.

    Fuck that guy, I thought. *What an asshole.*

    But after reading some of his reviews and of other eye doctors in the area, I started to reconsider. It had been almost two decades since the last time I saw him. I knew I definitely wasn't the same person I'd been back then. In all likelihood, he wasn't either. And though I couldn't see it as a teen, now I understood why he might've been so frustrated with me. Maybe it wasn't *him* who was the asshole back then – maybe it was *me*.

    I believe in giving second chances. People have bad days. Some people are just awful at making first impressions. And you never know what's going on in someone's life that makes them act the way they do. The cashier at the grocery store who was rude to you? Maybe her cat and sole companion in life just got run over by a Mack truck that morning. The guy who cut you off in traffic and then flipped *you* off?

Maybe he just caught his wife of twenty years banging the mailman. You never know why people act the way they do. Who knows, maybe the last person to be mean to you was grouchy because they have an invisible illness and were in a lot of pain that day. You just never know. So whenever I can, I always like to give people second chances. But I never, *ever* give thirds. There's a fine line between being nice and being a pushover.

Ultimately, I decided to give Dr. Masterson a second chance. All of his online reviews were positive and his office was only ten minutes from where I lived. I went in, the nurse dilated my pupils, and I waited for the doctor in his office. The eye drops she put in didn't bother me nearly as much as I remembered them bothering me as a teen. Don't get me wrong: they didn't feel great. But it certainly wasn't the end of the world.

Dr. Masterson came into the exam room before long. He looked a lot like I'd remembered him: bald and with glasses. That's all that came to mind when I tried to picture him. It had been nearly twenty years after all. But he looked like an older version of the bald, grumpy, spectacled eye doctor I'd met that one Saturday morning in my teens. This time, he wasn't so grumpy. In fact, he was polite, professional, and pleasant. Dr. Masterson was now in his sixties and moved slowly. His demeanor was calm and courteous. All things considered, he seemed like a good dude.

The eye exam was quick and painless. It's still not something I look forward to getting done, but it's not something I dread anymore. Dr. Masterson could still see the scarring in the retina of my left eye from when I was a teenager. But other than that, everything else was normal. Exactly what I wanted to hear.

I brought up the first time we'd met when I was a teenager – *after* the exam was over. If his memory of me was as negative as mine was of him, I didn't want it to influence his treatment of me. I didn't know what kind of unnecessary, sadistic procedure an ophthalmologist might have up his sleeve for a patient he disliked – and I didn't want to find out. As it turned out, Dr. Masterson couldn't recall much about our first meeting. Without being rude about it, I gave him a quick rundown of how I remembered things. Then I apologized to him for being my usual asshole-self back then. And in turn, he apologized to me. It was a nice moment.

Now I see Dr. Masterson or one of his colleagues every couple years to make sure there isn't any new inflammation in my eyes. He's always pleasant. And while I can't say I look forward to having my eyes dilated and examined, I do look forward to saying hi to Dr. Masterson and seeing what's new with the good doctor.

In addition to seeing an eye doctor, I also started regularly seeing a rheumatologist again. After that first appointment with Dr. Sack's associate, Dr. Schwartz, I began regularly seeing my old rheumy again. Dr. Sack, now deep into his seventies, looked good for his age and had the same compassionate personality I remembered from my teens and early twenties. I asked him if he ever planned to retire a couple of times and each time I got the same answer:

"I'll retire two weeks after I'm dead," Dr. Sack would say with a smile.

For years, I'd wanted to thank him for something. I thought about it every once in a while but didn't think I'd ever get the chance to tell him.

When the Behcet's decided to come out to play after years of remission forcing me to start seeing doctors again, I would have my chance.

"Well, Ellis," Dr. Sack said at the end of one of our appointments, offering me his hand, "it was nice to see you as always. Why don't you check back in with me in about six months. Of course, if you have any symptoms or need anything before then, don't hesitate to come see me."

"It was nice to see you, too. And I won't hesitate," I said, shaking the doctors hand. "There's just one more thing."

"What's that?" he asked, turning around, his hand already on the doorknob.

"I need to thank you for something. I've wanted to for a very long time."

Dr. Sack stepped away from the door and looked me in the eyes, giving me his full attention.

"As you know, all throughout my teens, I was in *a lot* of pain. Between the oral ulcers, the genital ulcers, the clots, and everything else, I was miserable. You were the only doctor who was willing to give me what I needed to get some relief. Those extra-strength Vicodin made life almost tolerable during those awful years. If it wasn't for those pills, I probably would've tried to kill myself a lot sooner than I did. The fact that I'd eventually have problems with them doesn't matter. I know the drug company that made Vicodin marketed it to doctors as a safer, much-less-addictive alternative to drugs like morphine and codeine. Now we all know that to be utter bullshit to which I can personally attest. But all you cared about was my comfort. You saw a scared teenage kid in a lot of pain and you wanted to help. And you did. So for that: thank you, doctor. Thank you so very, very much."

"I appreciate that," Dr. Sack said with a smile. "But you don't have to thank me. I'm just glad they helped."

We shook hands and he left the room, off to see his next patient. That was one of the last times I'd ever see Dr. Sack. He was killed in a car accident in January of 2018.

He retired two weeks later.

"Health is the crown on the well person's head that only the ill person can see." - Robin Sharma

27. Back In Action

The swelling and pain from the DVTs in my legs got progressively better over the summer of 2015. By my birthday in early August, I was mobile enough to go back to work. Of course, I waited until *after* my birthday to go back. But I went back shortly thereafter. My right leg still wasn't totally back to normal, but most of the swelling had gone down and I could be on it long enough to fulfill all my responsibilities. The first thing I did upon returning to work was sign up for short-term disability insurance. Fortunately, I'd had enough money saved up to be out of work for the three-or-so months I had been. But I could've stayed out for four or five if I'd had short-term disability.

When I returned to the overnight management job, the motivation to build my writing career was higher than ever. Being home for three months, being able to wake up whenever I felt like it, setting my own schedule, not having anyone other than myself to answer to – it was a taste of the life I could live year round if I worked hard for it. But my freshly renewed motivation wasn't just limited to my writing.

The clots in my legs and the pain in my stomach reminded me of the harsh reality of living with Behcet's disease. At any time I could become blind, deaf, paralyzed, or dead. That thought lights a fire under my ass, keeping me moving forward with everything I've got – while I've still got it. In addition to using that motivation for my writing, I wanted to start traveling more. I wanted to meet cool, interesting people and spend more time with all the awesome friends and family I already had in my life. And I wanted to get out there and start dating again.

After Steph and I broke up, I didn't date for years. Between the lingering devastation of our breakup and the depression I'd gone through, I didn't have the desire or energy to start seeing anyone. But by the time the clots hit, that'd changed. I'd already been out with a couple of women, but I decided to make dating more of a priority. I wasn't looking to settle down with anyone, but I do enjoy the company of women and like having someone to do stuff with. So I started putting myself out there more, making connections, and going out on dates. I could easily write a whole memoir about my dating experiences over the past few years. But this memoir is about living with Behcet's, so I'm only mentioning women who are relevant to *this* story. To hear the juicy gossip about all the others, you'll just have to read my dating memoir when it comes out.[1]

I was still taking Coumadin, the blood thinner, when I returned to work. Regular blood work is required when taking Coumadin to make sure your blood thickness[2] is within the normal range. They use a measurement called the International Normalized Ratio (INR). The results of each test would determine when I'd have to get checked again. If the INR came back within range, I wouldn't have to go back for a couple of weeks. But if it was too high or low, the doctor would adjust my Coumadin dosage and I'd

---

[1] I doubt I'll write such a memoir. However, I do intend to eventually write a memoir about my experience working with special-needs teens for fifteen years.

[2] Again, blood thinners don't actually thin your blood.

have to go back a day or two later. Some weeks I'd have to go to the lab as many as three-or-even-four times. For a procedure that only involved poking me in the arm, it sure was a huge pain in my ass.

The lab I had to get blood drawn from is about forty-five minutes from where I lived. While out of work, I really didn't mind going. I actually almost enjoyed it because it got me out of the house for a little while and I liked talking with the phlebotomists. But once back at work, taking time out of my day to get blood drawn quickly became a major inconvenience – especially when I had to do it several times in the same week.

I did some research and found out that they make home INR monitors. They work just like home glucose meters for people with diabetes. You prick your finger, squeeze a drop of blood onto the test strip, stick it in the machine, and voila! Within seconds, it gives you your INR.

I made an appointment with my primary care physician and brought him some literature and forms to fill out. You can only get the home INR machine with a doctor's order. We talked it over and he agreed I'd be an ideal candidate. He filled out the forms and my insurance approved it. A couple weeks later I had a very kind and informative woman at my home with the machine showing me how to use it.

That thing made my life soooooo much easier. It must've saved me dozens, if not hundreds of hours over the following months. Me, my PCP, and my rheumatologist all agreed I should stay on Coumadin for at least six-to-nine months. We even talked about the possibility of me staying on it indefinitely since more clots could form at any time. Of course, I didn't like the idea of having to take *any* drug for the rest of my life. But if doing so would prevent me from getting more blood clots, it was at least worth considering. The clots themselves, as inconvenient and painful as they might be, don't really pose any serious health risks – not directly. What the clots can lead to, however, is potentially *very* serious.

About twenty-five percent of Behcet's patients, mostly males, experience inflammation in their leg veins at some point. About five percent develop a clot in one of the deep veins in their legs.[1] As you know, I'm part of that unlucky five percent. But I haven't had *just one* deep-vein clot: I've had a number of DVTs. Any clot has the potential to turn deadly. Clots in the deep veins of the legs can dislodge and travel to the lungs, leading to pulmonary embolism (PE). If you don't know what that is, it ain't good. An embolism is a blockage in a blood vessel. A PE is when that blockage is in the lungs. As you might imagine, having blocked blood vessels in your lungs is something to be avoided. Pulmonary embolism can cause a number of problems, the most serious of which is sudden death. So you can see why the idea of staying on blood thinners indefinitely was being thrown around.

In the fall of 2015, I got back into hitting the gym at least four-or-five times a week. My legs were totally back to normal. For the first time since the clots I'd gotten in my teens, they even *looked* normal. No longer was my left calf a little bit larger than the other. The slight-but-permanent left-leg swelling that remained after the 1998 clots got balanced out by the slight-but-permanent right-leg swelling that lingered

---

[1] Behcet's syndrome and blood vessels. (2008). *Behcet's Syndrome Society*. Retrieved October 22, 2020 from https://behcetsuk.org/Documents/web%20blood%20vessels.pdf

after the 2015 clots. After having different-sized calves for nearly two decades, I was happy to finally get my symmetry back.

The 2015 clots also left some new varicose veins along my right leg and the right side of my abdomen. Those abdominal veins were right across from the ones on my left side and also gave me a more-symmetrical appearance. While I don't like the way they look, apparently I'm the only one. Like my other varicose veins, I've received compliments from women and men alike about them. I don't know what it is, but I'm not complaining. I'll take a compliment wherever I can get one.

Between the clots, being out of work, all the doctor appointments, all the trips to the lab to get blood work, the stomach pain on the Fourth of July, and everything else, 2015 was an eventful year – especially that summer. But by mid-autumn, things had calmed down considerably, including my illness. What *didn't* calm down at all was my spirit. For years I'd gotten complacent. Sure, I knew in the back of my mind that I had Behcet's disease. But since it'd been in remission, it wasn't something I spent much time thinking about. When the 2015 clots hit, I was forced to look my shitty illness right in the face for the first time in years. I stared it down long and hard, letting it fuel the fire burning inside me. It motivated me to live a little faster, love a little harder, laugh a little more, and chase my dreams with everything I've got.

And that's exactly what I did. For the next several years, I did a lot of traveling and a lot of dating, I worked even harder at my writing career so I could eventually quit my overnight job, I spent more quality time with my son and other family members, and just lived more fully in general. With the Behcet's motivating me to get out there and live but without any serious symptoms preventing me from actually doing so, I was going full throttle. But the Behcet's wasn't gone for good – it was just taking some time to rest so it could fuck me up all over again a couple years later.

"The past does not repeat itself, but it rhymes." - Mark Twain

28. Clot Again

After the clots and the stomach inflammation in the summer of 2015, I didn't have any serious Behcet's symptoms for the next couple of years. Everything was going good. My writing career was coming along nicely and my income was steadily increasing slowly but surely. I was consistently hitting the gym hard and had the body to show for it. Things were good with my son, my family, and my friends. I did a lot of traveling, disappearing every few months, usually to go someplace warm and sunny. And I had a very active social life, dating one wonderful woman after the next. Life was good.

I'd even come off Coumadin after being on it for close to eighteen months. The clots had long since dissolved and my legs were back to normal. Though my doctors and I had previously considered the possibility of staying on Coumadin permanently to prevent future clots, we all agreed that since more than fifteen years passed between the first series of clots and the second, it was unlikely that I'd develop more anytime soon.

We were all wrong.

Living with Behcet's disease has taught me a lot about probability. Just because something is unlikely doesn't mean it won't happen. It's incredibly unlikely that any given person in the USA will have Behcet's. Yet here I am. The odds of having Behcet's in the United States is about one in three-hundred thousand.[1] For men, the odds are even worse. Only about one in every four-hundred-thousand men have Behcet's in the US. Yet, once again, here I am. I thought about that a lot in the years following my diagnosis. Odds don't mean a thing when you're talking about any given person. The odds of getting struck by lightening or winning the lottery are overwhelmingly unlikely. Yet they both happen to people. Some people even win the lottery or get struck by lightening more than once. You never really know what's going to happen to *you*. Just like me and my doctors couldn't have known what was going to happen to *me*.

  In the late winter/early spring of 2018, after two-and-a-half years without any serious symptoms, I started having some mild stiffness and swelling in my left leg. Though I didn't think it was anything serious at first, I kept a close eye on things. Of course, it was on a Friday night that I first noticed the swelling. When I woke up the next day, my leg was much worse. The swelling had increased and my range of motion had decreased. I continued to monitor things closely and considered going to the emergency room, though I really didn't want to. All day Saturday my leg stayed the same, so I stayed home. I went to bed that night prepared to go to the ER Sunday morning if my leg got any worse. Fortunately, it didn't seem to be any worse when I woke up the next day. But it wasn't any better, either. So I decided to call my primary first thing Monday morning to set up an appointment. I called in sick to work Sunday night, the first time I'd been out since 2015, then called my

---

[1] Calamia, K., Wilson, F., Icen, M., Crowson, C., Gabriel, S., & Kremers, H. (2009). Epidemiology and clinical characteristics of Behcet's disease in the US: a population-based study. *Arthritis & Rheumatology*, 61(5):600-4.

doctor's office Monday morning. He was able to see me that afternoon. By then my leg was really starting to get sore. But the left was nowhere near as bad as I'd let my right leg get before going to the doctor in 2015.

"Ellis," Dr. Banerjee said as he entered the exam room. "What's troubling you?"

"I have more clots," I replied as I dropped my pants to show him the swollen leg. "It feels just like it did when I had the clots a few years ago. Looks like I'll need to go back on blood thinners."

"Let's get an ultrasound and see what's what first, okay?"

"I really don't want to have to be admitted to the hospital if I can help it," I said.

The doctor glanced at his watch and replied, "You might not have to. Let me call downstairs and see if they have room to squeeze you in."

Fortunately, they did. Dr. Banerjee's office was on the second floor of a large medical building. He ordered a stat ultrasound from radiology on the first floor and they got me in right away. Like my two previous ultrasound experiences, the technician was female. Three for three. It made me wonder if it's a female-dominated field. I certainly didn't have a problem if it was. In fact, if I had to have someone smearing gel all over me and slowly dragging a scanning device past my crotch, I'd rather it be a woman. As it turns out, as many as ninety-percent of sonographers are female.[1] Fun fact.

The woman who did my ultrasound was cool,

---

[1]   Is sonography a good career? Discover benefits and risks. (n.d.). *Ultrasound Technician Center.* Retrieved October 23, 2020 from https://www.ultrasoundtechniciancenter.org/jobs-and-careers/benefits-and-risks.html

just like the others I'd had over the years. She scanned both of my legs even though there was only pain and swelling in the left one, just like the last ultrasound technician had done in 2015. And just like in 2015, the ultrasound revealed multiple clots in *both* legs. The radiologist sent the results upstairs to Dr. Banerjee just minutes before he was getting ready to leave his office for the day. I went back upstairs for a quick consult with the doctor.

"Looks like you were right again," Dr. Banerjee said with a hint of surprise in his voice. "You've got massive clots in both legs."

"Yeah," I replied. "The radiologist told *me* just like I told *you*. I've been living with Behcet's disease for decades, doctor. I know what it feels like when the blood vessels in my legs get inflamed. And I not only know what it feels like when clots form, I know what objective signs and symptoms to look for."

"I know you do, Ellis," Dr. Banerjee replied. "It's not that I doubted you. But there are certain-"

"Protocols, rules, regulations, and everything else," I interrupted. "I know, I know. I'm sorry if I came across as rude. It's just frustrating for me sometimes, as I know it is for you, too." I glanced down at my watch. It was five-o-clock on the dot. "I also know you're trying to get out of here and you're doing me a favor by seeing me when you could've sent me to the ER. So I don't want to take up any more of your time than necessary."

"I appreciate that. So the question is: what do we do now? I could prescribe you subcutaneous heparin injections and Coumadin like they gave you in the hospital the last time you had clots."

"Or?" I asked, sensing there was more to

come.

"Or we could try one of the newer blood thinners that have come on the market over the past few years."

"I'll need to do more research," I replied, "but I've read a little bit about some of the newer blood thinners and I like what I've learned so far. Consistent dosing, no blood work-"

"Exactly."

"What do *you* think?" I asked. "What's your experience with them? I know there are several of them on the market: Xarelto, Pradaxa-"

"In general, I think they're great – a big improvement over older blood thinners for the reasons you just mentioned. For you, I would suggest Eliquis."

"Let's go with Eliquis then."

"Alright," Dr. Banerjee replied, then immediately got to work sending the electronic prescription over to my pharmacy. As doctors often do, he continued talking to me while his attention was focused on the computer, his fingers typing away swiftly. "You're going to take two tablets twice a day for five days. Then you're going to go down to taking one tablet twice a day and stay at that dose. I want you to come back and see me in a week. But if your leg gets worse or you experience any new symptoms, come see me before then."

"Understood," I said. Dr. Banerjee finished typing, swung around in his chair to face me, stood up, and offered me his hand. As I shook it, I said, "Thank you, doctor. Enjoy your evening."

"You too," he replied, smiled, and disappeared out the door.

And just like that, I was back on blood

thinners. But this time, I didn't have to get any blood work done. I'd returned the home INR monitor many months earlier. So if I'd gone back on Coumadin, I would've had to start going back to the lab. And that would've been a huge pain in the ass. As always, I did a lot of research into Eliquis before taking it and decided it was worth a try. Aside from some mild nausea for the first few week I was on it, I didn't have any side effects. Once the dose switched from four pills a day to just two, the nausea pretty much disappeared.

After going to the doctor, getting the ultrasound, and picking up the Eliquis prescription, I headed home to get some rest. I should've called in sick to work that night like I'd done the night before. Or what I *really* should've done, I should've gotten a note from my doctor and taken a few weeks off to fully recover. After all, that's the point of paying for short-term disability insurance like I'd been doing since returning to work after being out with the clots last time. But I didn't do that. Foolishly, I went into work that night. Maybe it was out of pride. Or maybe out of a sense of responsibility. I knew that they were already short staffed. Me being out would've have a negative impact on the teens directly under my care and made the jobs of my two supervisors – both of whom I considered friends – harder. So even though I didn't get much rest during the day, I went into work that night.

But I really, *really* wish I hadn't.

It was mid-March and there was a blizzard that night, dropping over half-a-foot of snow on the ground. In the mornings after waking the students up, I had to feed them, give them their medications (or *fedicate* them, as I liked to call it), and then walk them to class. The residence I managed was on one side of the campus and I had to bring some of my students to the other side, which was about a quarter-mile away. The campus itself was quite beautiful, especially with all the fresh snow on the ground, in the trees, and on top of all the buildings. Normally I enjoyed walking the student to class. But having to walk a half-mile through six inches of snow with swollen, clot-filled legs was anything but enjoyable.

No one at work knew about the clots. I didn't tell either of my supervisors, any staff, and certainly not any of the students. I'm supposed to have at least one other staff working with me, but I didn't that night. Otherwise, I could've had them transition the student to class. But I was by myself which meant I had no choice but to bring them to class myself. Every single step that morning was agony. Having to lift my stiff, heavy, sore left leg over and over to get through the snow was torturous. But I kept the suffering to myself and no one suspected anything was wrong.

The rest of that work week was no better. Every morning as I walked the students to school, in my head I was thinking the same thing:

I should've called in sick. Actually, what I really should've done was get a note from my doctor and gone out on disability for a month or two. But oh no. I didn't do that. I decided, for whatever stupid reason, to go into work like nothing's wrong. Why do I do this to myself?

Since we were so short staffed, I had to work alone that whole week. It sucked. The mornings when I had to walk the students to school did, anyway. But I got through through the week. And by the time the weekend finally arrived, the Eliquis had started working. The pain and swelling in my left leg was slowly starting to get better.

"Sometimes you just have to live your life, even if that means letting go of someone who meant the world to you." - Unknown

29. Breaking Up

I'm glad my doctor and I decided to give Eliquis a try. I'm still on it to this day and like it a lot better than Coumadin. After talking it over with my primary care physician and rheumatologist, we all agreed I should probably stay on a blood thinner indefinitely. This was the third time the inflammation in my blood vessels led to clots. And without staying on a blood thinner, it likely wouldn't be the last. So I've stayed on Eliquis and, aside from the drug's high price tag, I haven't had any problems with it.

My left leg slowly got better in the weeks after starting Eliquis. At the time, I was dating an awesome young woman named Daisy who I'd met the summer before. When we first started seeing each other, she had an apartment in East Providence which wasn't too far from me. Daisy was doing part of an internship there after getting her doctorate in optometry. But the last part of her internship was in South Carolina. I'd helped her move down there a couple of weeks before the clots formed on what was one of the best road trips of my life – and I'm a road trip veteran with plenty of amazing adventures under my belt. I was planning to fly back down there to visit her at the end of March. When the clots happened, I became worried that it might affect my trip.

It's no secret that long flights can cause blood clots in some people. But what isn't well known is whether or not it's safe to fly in the weeks after getting clots. Some doctors recommend waiting at least four weeks before flying. My flight was scheduled for just two weeks after the clots formed. I did some research and even though I'd already made up my mind, I asked my doctor for his opinion. He confirmed the conclusion I'd already come to: that in all likelihood it would be fine. So about a week into the spring of 2018, I flew from Boston to Columbia, South Carolina to visit my girlfriend.

My leg was feeling a lot better than it'd felt a couple weeks earlier, but it was still far from being back to normal. Daisy knew about the clots. I was up front with her about having Behcet's disease from the beginning. She was the only woman I'd ever dated who had heard of it. Since eye problems are one of the disease's main symptoms, Daisy had learned about it in optometry school. Like every other eye doctor I've met, Daisy had a prescription for glasses and contacts. She also had two of the biggest, most beautiful blue eyes I'd ever seen. Ass and eyes – they get me every time. If it's not one, it's the other. And Daisy had both. As soon as I met her, between the brains, the butt, and the big, beautiful blues, I knew she had me.

Getting to Columbia was fine. During a layover in Virginia, I had to practically run from one side of the airport to the other so I wouldn't miss the plane. My first flight had been delayed which only left me a few minutes to get from one terminal to the other. But I made it – and just in the nick of time.

When I boarded that second flight, my leg was just starting to hurt from speed walking my way across the airport. Fortunately, I was seated in the last row of the small American Airlines Airbus with no one in the seat next to me and I had plenty of room to stretch out. It was a short flight from Arlington, VA to Columbia, SC and my leg felt better by the time we landed.

My girlfriend picked me up at the airport and we went out to dinner. When Daisy asked how my leg was doing, I told her it was much better and almost back to normal. It *was* much better than it had been even a week earlier and it *was* gradually getting a little closer to being back to normal with every passing day. But I definitely downplayed how much it still hurt when I had to be on it for long periods of time. I had too much respect for Daisy to flat-out lie. But I also didn't want to come across as weak or seeming like I was looking for any kind of special treatment. Plus, I didn't want her to worry about me.

Over the next few days, my time was spent doing one of two things. Either I'd be lounging around Daisy's apartment where we'd be watching shows and movies, enjoying some delicious South Carolina cuisine, kissing and cuddling under the covers, relaxing, and enjoying each other's company. Or I'd be out and about with Daisy exploring the city of Columbia and the surrounding area.

On the third day I was down there, Daisy took me to Sesquicentennial State Park. Her and I both enjoyed being outdoors and had gone on several nature walks in the past. There was a small lake in the middle of the park and we walked all the way around it: roughly two miles. The terrain was mostly flat and it wasn't too hard on my leg. However, I did have to stop a couple of times – but only for a minute here, a minute there. After being on it for a while, my left leg would swell up and start to feel a little uncomfortable. But I just needed to get off it for a minute or two and then I could resume walking.

Daisy and I made it all the way around the

lake. Though I was honest with her about my leg getting sore, I downplayed just how sore it actually was. At times it really hurt. But a short rest was all I needed before I could keep going.

  They had paddle boats and canoes you could rent to take out on the lake. We wanted to rent a paddle boat, but they didn't have any available. So we rented a canoe and a couple of life jackets instead. It had been over a decade since the last time I'd been in a canoe, but I remembered everything I needed to know to safely use it. After we had our vests on and Daisy got in the front, I pushed off, hopped in the back, and off we went. Her and I paddled around the lake for a while. It was beautiful and gave me some time off my feet.

  Walking around Sesquicentennial State Park gave me a much-needed confidence boost. I'd been worried about doing any kind of physical activity that required being on my feet for more than a few minutes. Even though my leg swelled up a bit and I did have to stop a few times, it wasn't nearly as bad as I was afraid it could've been.

  Daisy and I had talked about going for a long walk along the Columbia Canal. But we agreed it'd be best to wait and see how well I was able to tolerate walking around Sesquicentennial State Park first. Since the hike around the lake went well, I felt confident I'd be able to hike along the canal without much of a problem.

  As it turned out, the walk along the Columbia Canal was a lot rougher than the walk around Sesquicentennial State Park. Not only was it a lot longer of a walk, it was also much hillier. Daisy and I got to the canal in the late morning. It was seventy-five degrees and sunny – perfect weather – just like it had been the previous few days since I'd arrived in South Carolina. But a bittersweet mood lingered between Daisy and I.

As nice as it was outside and as much as I enjoyed spending time with her, I knew that Daisy would only be my girlfriend for a few more hours until she dropped me off at the airport in the late evening. Before leaving for the canal, her and I had a long talk that morning. She's more than a decade younger than me and we were at different points in our lives. Daisy had just gotten her doctorate and was wrapping up an internship so she could get full licensure as an optometrist. As soon as that was all taken care of, she wanted to find someone to settle down and have kids with.

Now don't get me wrong: I love my son more than anything in the world. If it wasn't for him, in all likelihood I wouldn't be alive today. But I don't want any more children. Not anytime soon, anyway. Probably not ever – but you never know. Life takes some weird twists and turns sometimes and you find yourself considering things you never in a million years thought you ever would've. So I generally never say never.

That being said...

I never wanted kids to begin with, if I'm being honest. My son wasn't planned – it just sort of happened. And again, him being born turned out to be the greatest thing that's ever happened to me. But I'm one-hundred-percent positive I don't want any more kids for the foreseeable future. In fact, I've actually considered getting a vasectomy. That's how badly I don't want any more kids right now – enough to let some dude cut into my scar-covered balls. Not only would having more children seriously complicate my career-building-and-world-traveling plans. There's another factor to consider: Behcet's disease. What if I passed it on to my next child? Or what if my own illness ravaged my body so badly that I couldn't be even a half-decent father? The only way to make sure those things don't happen is to not have any more kids.

 My son just turned thirteen in May. It's hard to believe I'm the forty-year-old father of a teenager. Fortunately – and I thank the universe every single day for this – he hasn't shown a single sign of having Behcet's disease. By the time I was thirteen, I had sores all over me, crippling stomach pain, extreme fatigue, and other symptoms. My son has none and I couldn't be more thankful. But if I had another child, s/he might not be so lucky.

 Daisy and I walked along the Columbia Canal, hand in hand, knowing it was likely the last time we'd see each other – for a very long time at least. We followed the canal for over two miles. The view was absolutely breathtaking. It was the first week of spring and we saw a lot of different animals out and about for the first time since the fall. There were also a lot of other people out walking along the canal, many with their children and pets. My leg wasn't bothering me too badly for the first mile-and-a-half-or-so. But by the time we'd walked two miles, it was getting stiff and starting to swell. I would've liked to have followed the canal a bit farther, but suggested we turn around shortly after the two-mile mark.

 As we started walking back the way we came, it dawned on me that we'd been walking at a decline the entire time. The walk back was all uphill, though the incline was slight for most of the way. Slight as it was, it still caused my leg to start hurting before long.

I did everything I could to keep going, hiding my discomfort from Daisy. If our impending breakup hadn't been just a few short hours away, I wouldn't've tried to hide how sore my leg had been feeling. But I didn't want her final memories of us together to include me bitching and complaining about my leg. So I sucked it up as best I could and kept going.

Eventually, maybe one-third of the way back, the pain became unbearable. The old me would've concocted some ridiculous lie to hide the true cause of my pain. But that was the old me. The new me accepted the fact that I had Behcet's disease. Besides, Daisy wouldn't have believed me if I told her it was from a skateboarding accident or something similarly preposterous. Daisy's one smart cookie and would've seen right through that bullshit. But more importantly, I didn't want to lie to her. So as hard as it was for me to do, I told Daisy the truth.

"I need to sit down for a couple of minutes," I said.

"Your leg bothering you?" Daisy asked, genuine concern in her voice.

"I'll be fine," I replied. "I just need to rest it for a minute."

"I had a feeling your leg was bothering you more than you were letting on," she said. "If your leg's hurting, you should've said you wanted to turn around sooner. I would've understood. You know that. At least I'd like to think you know me well enough to know that."

See? Smart cookie.

"You're right: I *do* know that," I replied, taking Daisy's hand in mine as she sat down next to me on the bench. "And I'd like to think that *you* know *me* well enough to know that I don't let this illness stop me from doing what I want to do. And I wanted to at least make it down to the bridge, which we did."

"I just don't want you to feel like you need to try to impress me."

"I don't," I replied with a smirk. "I know I *already* impress the shit out of you – and that's without even trying."

"Wow," Daisy said with a half-smile, shaking her head. "You're still cocky even when you're in pain."

"And you're still sexy when you're pretending that you don't love how confident I am."

"How *cocky* you are," Daisy corrected with a smirk.

"I'll show *you* cocky when we get back to your apartment," I replied, pulling Daisy in for a kiss.

We got up and continued walking a minute later. My leg started hurting again before long, but I pushed through the pain until it once again became unbearable. I hoped to make it back to the car but needed to take one more break. We sat down for another couple minutes, then continued walking along the canal until we got back to the parking lot. By the time I got in her car, my leg was killing me again. My left thigh and calf were so swollen they felt like they were made of metal. But the swelling and pain gradually went down as we left the Columbia Canal and headed back to Daisy's apartment.

My leg was fine for the rest of the day. Though I hadn't wanted Daisy to see me in pain like that, I was glad we went for the canal walk. She'd told me before we left in the morning that she'd understand if I wanted to do something that required less walking. But I wanted to see the canal and am glad that I did.

After going back to Daisy's apartment to enjoy our last few hours of alone time together, she brought me to the airport. We stood outside at the departure-drop-off area hugging and kissing for what probably seemed like an eternity to anyone watching us, but it never could've been long enough for me. I wiped the tears from Daisy's gorgeous blue eyes, gave her one last kiss on the lips, grabbed my stuff, and headed into the airport. And that was the last time I ever laid *my* eyes on that amazing woman.

I've dated a lot of wonderful women in the years since Steph and I broke up. But none of them made me question what I want out of life nearly as much as Daisy. That girl really made me reconsider my priorities. If I'd wanted more kids, if I'd wanted to settle down and start a family, Daisy would've made an ideal partner. There's no doubt in my mind that she's going to be a great mother. And for some very lucky guy, she's going to make an amazing wife. But that guy won't be me. Not in 2018, not now, and probably not ever.

But I never say *never*.

Maybe five years from now I decide that I *do* want more kids. Is it likely? Nope. But is it possible? Sure. Stranger things have certainly happened. There were things I was 100% sure of ten years ago that I now know to be 100% false. Opinions change. Plans change. And that's why I eventually ruled out getting a vasectomy: because you never know what the future will bring. But for now, I don't want any more mini-mes running around.

After Daisy dropped me off at the Columbia airport, I flew back to Boston. The next few weeks were a bit rough, but not because of my leg. That was still steadily getting better as the clots continued to break up. But I wondered if I'd made the right decision about Daisy. To this day, I still think about it from time to time. Ultimately, whenever I do, I always come to the same conclusion: we did what was best for both of us. But fuck, do I miss that woman.

"Only through our connectedness to others can we really know and enhance the self. And only through working on the self can we begin to enhance our connectedness to others." - Harriet Goldhor Lerner

30. Olivia

To get over a breakup as quickly as possible, people often jump right into a new relationship – a rebound relationship. It's a tactic I've successfully employed on occasion over the years myself. But after Daisy and I broke up, I decided to stay away from women for a few months. I'd liked Daisy a lot and wanted to give myself time to miss her. And miss her I did. But after giving it two-or-three months, I got back out there and started dating again. And for the better part of the next year, I'd always be dating someone. But then in early 2019, after breaking up with a wonderful social worker I'd been seeing for a few months, I made the decision to stay single for a while – a long while.

Dating is a lot of fun. It's also a lot of work. Maintaining relationships take time and effort, the exact two things needed to build a successful writing career. It occurred to me that the time and energy I was putting into dating would've been better spent being channeled into my work. Dating is great and I love spending time with women – but it's distracting. So I decided to stop dating indefinitely to focus more on my writing career.

And that's what I did. But I didn't stop talking to women entirely. I still had a lot of female friends – guys, too – who I'd chat with online and occasionally get together with in person. As introverted as I can often be, I'm not asocial. I do like talking to and spending time with people, even if it's only online.

In addition to chatting with existing friends, I also made some new ones in the months following my decision to take a break from dating. One of them was a woman named Olivia who I'd met on Facebook in a Behcet's disease group that May. She sent me a friend request, I accepted it, and we began chatting regularly.

Olivia and I hit it off immediately. She's from New Jersey and grew up in the same town I'd visited to go to Wrestlemania 35 with my brother just a week before we started talking. Small world. Initially, it was our Behcet's diagnoses that brought us together. But as we got to know each other a little bit, we realized we had a lot more than just our shitty illnesses in common. For one, Olivia enjoyed weed as much as I did. Like me, she used cannabis for both recreational and medicinal purposes. THC and CBD, two compounds found in cannabis, work great at reducing the severity of several Behcet's symptoms. Joint and muscle pain, anxiety, upset stomach, insomnia: these are just a few examples. THC and CBD also work great at reducing the severity of side effects from the prescription drugs used to treat the symptoms of Behcet's. For example, the nausea I'd sometimes get from being on azathioprine and Eliquis could be reversed with a small dose of good ol' vitamin THC. And as an added benefit on top of its medicinal properties, weed just makes you feel good. It makes everything a little better: food tastes yummier, music is more enjoyable, comedy is funnier, and life doesn't seem so damn serious all the time.

If you haven't tried cannabis, I *high*ly recommend it.

Behcet's and bud weren't the only things Olivia and I bonded over. We both had the same nothing's-off-limits sense of humor, something that can only be developed through hardship as a way to deal with the pain. Battle-hardened soldiers often develop it after being deployed. If they weren't able to laugh at the absurdity and horrors of war, they'd go mad. First responders get it, too. When I was an EMT, we all developed what most people would consider a sick, morbid sense of humor. But it's practically a job requirement. Responding to calls where you regularly see bones sticking out of people's bodies, children getting permanently injured, teenagers dropping like flies from overdoses, and sometimes even worse, you need to learn to laugh about it. If you don't, the stress will – sooner or later – drive you bonkers. Living with a chronic illness can be the same way, especially one as painful as Behcet's. Many of us learn to see the humor in our dreadful conditions. If you can't learn to laugh about having a crotch full of ulcers – at least at times – your journey is going to be that much harder.

Olivia and I bonded over our diagnoses, love of weed, shared sense of humor, and more. We began messaging regularly, often daily. We talked about all kinds of things, from the foods we ate to the ulcers we'd get on our genitals. Before long, one particular topic started coming up and it came up often: sex. It'd been months since I'd been with anyone, so I was hornier than usual – and that's saying something. Even when I'd been on antidepressants years earlier, none of them ever put a dent in my libido.[1] Olivia had

---

[1] Antidepressants, particularly SSRIs, are notorious for causing sexual side effects. See: Higgins, A., Nash, M., & Lynch, A. (2010). Antidepressant-associated sexual dysfunction: impact,

just broken up with her boyfriend not too long before we'd met and was also experiencing heightened horniness. So it became a frequent topic of conversation, one we both very much enjoyed talking about.

But we didn't just *talk* about sex. Olivia and I began flirting, sending each other dirty pics. I hadn't sent dick pics to a lot of women in the past, but a few at least. However, Olivia was the first woman I could send them to without having to double check each pic to make sure you couldn't see the scars on my balls. With Olivia, I didn't care if they were visible. She already knew they were there because we'd talked about them plenty of times. Olivia had her own set of scars down there. It was incredibly freeing not having to worry, not having to even *think* about stuff like that. I might not have been overly self-conscious about having Behcet's disease like I was in my teens and twenties, but I still had to put thought into how to go about explaining it to the people I allowed into my life. With Olivia, I didn't have to explain shit. It was great.

Her and I continued to message often over the course of the summer of 2019. I'd made it clear to Olivia that I wasn't dating and wouldn't be for quite a while because I needed to stay focused on my work. The last thing I wanted to do was lead her on. But she was fine with keeping things casual: just two friends with the same shitty illness who enjoyed talking dirty to each other. Fresh out of a relationship with the father of her daughter, Olivia wasn't looking for anything serious either. It worked out perfectly for

---

effects, and treatment. *Drug, Healthcare, and Patient Safety*, 2:141-50.

both of us. And that's not even taking into consideration the fact that we lived more than two-hundred miles apart. So we each enjoyed having the other to talk to and flirt with from afar. Not only was it nice to have someone with Behcet's to flirt and exchange dirty pics with, it was just nice having someone else with the disease to regularly talk to. I'd made plenty of friends who had Behcet's in online groups, but none I'd gotten as close to or talked to as regularly as Olivia. She became my Behcet's bestie – her term – or Behcestie for short.

That fall after several months of talking online, Olivia and I decided to get together for a couple of days. She was living in Pennsylvania at the time. We picked a town about halfway between the two of us to meet: Waterbury, Connecticut. It's a small city of about 100,000 people in western Connecticut, roughly a two-hour drive for each of us. I'd never been there before. Originally, Olivia had suggested Hartford. But I'd already been to Hartford a few times and wanted to go someplace new, so I suggested Waterbury. Olivia was cool with it. I always enjoy exploring new places, so I looked forward to checking out Waterbury. I was even more eager to check Olivia out.

She got to Waterbury first. I arrived shortly thereafter. Olivia was waiting for me on a bench in the middle of the Waterbury Green. It was a warm early fall day and there were plenty of other people out and about. The green is a large, open grassy area with benches, a fifteen-foot-tall clock tower, and two war monuments, one at each end. Surrounding the green on all sides are old multi-story buildings that were factories once upon a time. For someone like me who grew up in New England, Waterbury is remarkably unremarkable. It reminded me of every other small city in the northeast. I might as well have been on the Taunton Green near where I grew up. They're both old factory cities. Taunton was once known at the Silver City, while Waterbury used to produce nearly half of the country's brass. The only difference between the two New England cities is the roads. Waterbury's roads are, well, good. Taunton's roads – if you can call them that – are mostly just potholes with some pavement between them. I've been all over this country and I've never seen worse roads anywhere. Unless you drive a dune buggy, I don't recommend joy riding around Taunton, Massachusetts.

    After finding somewhere to park, I approached my black-and-white-polka-dotted-dress-wearing Behcestie sitting on a bench in the middle of the Waterbury Green. Olivia had on a pair of black sunglasses and looked like Jackie O from afar. When she saw me coming, Olivia hopped up to her feet. We exchanged a hug, then sat down on the bench together. I could tell Olivia was a little nervous. Me? Cool as a cucumber. This wasn't the first time I'd met someone new in an unfamiliar place. I was a veteran online dater after all, though I'd deactivated the dating apps from my phone months earlier. Doing my best to make Olivia feel comfortable, we talked for a little while in the middle of the green. It seemed to work. Before long, we were joking and laughing about how quaint-yet-creepy the Waterbury looked.

    Olivia and I were both hungry and walked to a small hole-in-the-wall restaurant a few minutes from the green. She ordered a salad. I got salmon with curly fries. I'd had them each individually a thousand times before but never together. Turns out, it's a good combo. I enjoyed my food and Olivia enjoyed hers. We continued to talk for a while after finishing our lunches, going back and forth trading Behcet's war stories. She's only a few years younger than I am and had been diagnosed more recently than me, getting her first symptom in 2008, which is good news for her. Generally, the earlier in life Behcet's is diagnosed, the worse the prognosis. And Behcet's is usually more severe in men than it is in women.[1] Once again: lucky me.

After lunch, Olivia and I checked in at the hotel we'd booked. Our fifth-floor room was really nice. We relaxed for a little while, then I rolled us up a joint and we took a walk. The entire hotel was non-smoking, so we went up to the top of its five-story parking garage and sparked it up. The view of downtown Waterbury was pretty. So was Olivia. Once we were done smoking, her and I went back to the room.

I won't give you a play-by-play of what happened when we got back to the room. Or later that night. Or again the next morning. What I will say is that Olivia and I both had a really good time. I told her about how I'd always fantasized about hooking up with a woman who had Behcet's. She was happy to turn that fantasy into reality. I gave her a tour of all the wonderful scars the disease had left me over the years, from my face to my legs – and, of course, in between them. Olivia returned the favor and showed me hers. I'd never pointed out the scars on my balls to anyone without MD after their name before. Other

---

[1] Ucar-Comlekoglu, D., Fox, A., & Sen, H. (2014). Gender differences in Behcet's disease associated uveitis. *Journal of Ophthalmology*. Retrieved October 19, 2020 from https://www.hindawi.com/journals/joph/2014/820710/

women had noticed them – not many, but a few – and I explained their cause as best I could. With Olivia, I didn't have to. She already knew what caused them: the same thing that caused *her* scars.

Olivia and I bonded over our mutual pain and embarrassment. Even though we'd only just met in person, I felt an intimacy with her I never have with any other woman – or any other person, for that matter. And the satisfaction I got from turning a nearly-twenty-year-old fantasy into reality was off the charts. I wish I could go back and tell my twenty-year-old self that someday there'd be online groups of people with Behcet's to connect with and that I'd end up in bed with one of them. Maybe I would've felt better knowing my loneliness had an expiration date. For years, I thought I was destined to feel alone forever, like I was the only one on the planet with Behcet's. Getting the clots in 2015 and discovering Behcet's disease Facebook groups made me realize I wasn't alone. But it wasn't until I met Olivia in 2019 that I actually *felt* like I wasn't alone.

Before Olivia, there's only one other person I can recall meeting who *claimed* to have the diagnosis. It was way back in 1998 when I'd been hospitalized with my first clots. The guy who wheeled me from my second-floor room to radiology in the basement of Morton Hospital for what turned out to be an ultra-awkward-and-strangely-arousing ultrasound told me he also had Behcet's disease. But I was suspicious then and I still am now.

"You're just a kid," the twenty-something-year-old said as he pushed me down the hallway. "What are you here for?"

"An ultrasound, I guess," I replied. "Whatever that is."

"I know *that*. I'm the one bringing you. I mean why are you here at Morton?"

"Oh. They say I've got Behcet's syndrome or disease or something."

"Behcet's, huh? I've got that," he said as if it's as common as the flu. "Well, here we are. Good luck, kid."

"Yeah, thanks."

That was the extent of our conversation. Something about how casually he claimed to have Behcet's never sat right with me. My seventeen-year-old bullshit detector went off then and my forty-year-old one is going off thinking about it now. You don't just throw out that you have Behcet's like it's no big deal.

It *is* a big deal.

To this day, I have no idea if that guy was telling the truth. I'm not even sure who he was: a nurse, an orderly, a janitor, or just some dude who just happened to be walking by at the right time and offered to wheel me to radiology – I'll never know. What I *do* know is that Olivia was the first person I'd ever met who I was *sure* had Behcet's. Like me, she's got the scars to prove it.

After spending a couple of days having fun together in Connecticut, Olivia and I said goodbye. I haven't seen her since then, but we're still good friends and chat regularly. We've talked about the possibility of another meet up at some point, maybe going to a Behcet's disease conference together. I'm already looking forward to the next time I get to see my Behcestie.

"In order to carry a positive action we must develop here a positive vision." - Dalai Lama

31. 2020 Vision

2020 has been a strange year for all of us. But it's also been a great year for *me*. For starters, I haven't had any more serious Behcet's symptoms. Aside from some achy joints and a few minor skin issues like the small patch of cystic acne I currently have on my back, nothing.[1] I'm still taking the same medications I've been on for the past few years and my blood work continues to come back normal. I saw an ophthalmologist a couple months ago (not Dr. Masterson but an associate of his[2]) to make sure there'd been no new inflammation in my eyes. All good.

When the coronavirus pandemic began, I was still working overnights. But I'd stepped down from my management position and cut back to just three nights a week six-months earlier. All the hard work I'd put into my new career was starting to pay off. After being at it for five years, I was making more from my writing than from my overnight job. So I cut back on my hours with the plan of quitting for good on my fortieth birthday. But when the pandemic hit, I saw an opportunity to leave four-months sooner.

A lot of the residential students I worked with

---

[1] I did get a golf-ball-sized cyst on my jaw in 2019, the first that big in over twenty years. I was put on doxycycline and it gradually shrunk. Beginning to end, it was there for about five months.

[2] Like every other eye doctor I've met, she wears glasses. Maybe there *is* something to my silly theory after all. Nah, probably not.

went home during the early pandemic months and my employer had a reduced need for staff. They were cutting people's hours, many of whom were good friends of mine and couldn't afford to lose the money. I volunteered to go out on indefinite leave so they wouldn't have to cut back so many people's hours. My employer agreed and it allowed several friends to keep their normal schedules. Originally, I was going to take the time off unpaid. Then the federal government passed a bill that allowed workers with certain medical conditions and a doctor's note to go on *paid* leave.

It wasn't hard to get a note from one of my doctors. It was so easy, in fact, that I ended up getting notes from *two* of them. Between the Behcet's diagnosis and the immunosuppressant I'm on, the two doctors I happened to have appointments with around that time were both happy to write me a note. I submitted them to the human resources director at my job and just like that I was on a ten-week paid vacation.

I was diagnosed with Behcet's disease almost twenty-five years ago. During that time, my illness has cost me quite a bit of money: co-pays, hospital bills, medications, etc. But I've never benefited from it. Not financially. Between the restricted blood flow to my legs from all the inflammation and clots, the blurred vision in my eye, the ringing in my ears, and some other permanent gifts Behcet's has left me, I could've gone on disability a long time ago. But I've always chosen not to. It's not that I have anything against disability. I certainly don't judge anyone who's on it. It's just not for me. However, when the opportunity to get ten weeks of paid leave fell into my lap, I decided to finally make a little money from my shitty illness. The timing was perfect.

    My paid leave started around the beginning of April. Within the first couple weeks of being out, I decided that I wouldn't be going back. Since I was planning to quit the first week of August, it didn't make sense to. The paid leave would run out mid-June, leaving just a few weeks before my fortieth birthday. So I burned through the ten weeks of paid leave, put in my two weeks notice, and put in a request to use up the remainder of my paid time off (PTO). I had just enough PTO to cover the two weeks notice. As of the first of July, after fifteen years of service, I left the residential school I'd been working at since finishing my undergraduate degree in 2005.

    I can't even begin to tell you how satisfying these past few months have been. I'd been dreaming about quitting my job ever since I started writing professionally in July of 2014.[3] Actually doing it was unbelievably liberating. It took six years of working my fucking ass off day and night – literally day and night – but I did it. All the hard work, all the sacrifices I've had to make, all the blood, sweat, and tears: it's all been worth it. Now I get to set my own schedule, work *when*ever I want from *where*ver I want, and choose what projects to spend my time on. It's soooooo nice not having to wake up to an alarm everyday. I get up whenever I feel like it. I go to sleep whenever I feel like it. It's fucking great.

    My health – both mental and physical – has definitely improved since I quit my overnight job. Even though I've always been a night owl, working third shift got harder and harder with each passing

---

[3] I started writing on July 1, 2014, exactly six years to the day before officially leaving my job.

year. And it's terrible for you. It can affect everything from your mood to your hormones, your relationships to your stress levels. And of course your sleep. After six years of working overnights and having to sleep during the day half the week, it's nice to get to sleep at night *every* night. I have more energy during the day, my mood is better, I feel less stressed, and even my blood pressure is lower.

Now that I'm self-employed, I have to pay for my own health insurance. With Behcet's disease, insurance is a must. As much as I hate HMOs and the whole health-insurance system at large, it's not going to change anytime soon and I can't go without coverage. Fortunately, I live in a state that makes it easy and affordable for self-employed people to get health insurance. There are a lot of things I dislike about Massachusetts' politics, but healthcare isn't one of them. In fact, Massachusetts is ranked number one out of all-fifty states when it comes to healthcare.[1] I was easily able to find an affordable plan that covers all the specialists I see and all the medications I'm on.

Even though I had the luxury of sleeping and working whenever I wanted after leaving my job, it didn't take long to fall into a daily routine. All spring and summer I'd wake up around eight in the morning – give or take an hour – and immediately caffeinate. As soon as my brain started booting up, I'd get to work on my writing and whatever business-related tasks I had scheduled for that day. If it was raining outside I'd work deep into the afternoon, putting in at least an eight-hour day. But if it was nice out, I'd <u>work until the early afternoon</u> and then go do

---

[1] McCann, A. (2020, Aug. 3). Best & worst states for health care. *WalletHub*. Retrieved October 28, 2020 from https://wallethub.com/edu/states-with-best-health-care/23457

something outdoorsy.

After the coronavirus pandemic hit and entire industries were shut down, a lot of people spent the summer complaining about everything they couldn't do. No concerts, no festivals, no Fourth of July celebrations, no traveling, and no end to the shutdown in sight. Sure, I was bummed that the concerts I wanted to go to got canceled and that I wouldn't be seeing my friends on the Fourth. But I didn't focus on the negative, on what I *couldn't* do. I focused on what I *could*. And what I could do was spend a lot of time out in nature. So every nice afternoon I'd head to the beach to swim, surf, and soak up some sun, go kayaking and/or fishing at a nearby lake, or go for a long, socially-distanced nature walk with a friend. All things considered, I had a wicked good summer.

Now that it's fall, I'm spending more time indoors. I don't like it. I need sun and sand, warmth and water. Every year, I get a touch of seasonal depression and have for as long as I can remember. Some years it's bad, some years it's barely noticeable. In my teens and twenties I'd let it get to me, constantly complaining about the long, dark, cold New England winter months. That negative-ass attitude only made things worse. It'll do that. But the new-and-improved me sees things differently. As challenging as it can be sometimes, I try to maintain a positive attitude year round. Instead of getting caught up in negativity, focusing on how much the winter sucks, I channel my energy into positive things. Over the past several years since starting my writing career, I've taken on more projects and worked longer hours in the fall and winter. This serves two purposes. One, it allows me to work less in the spring and summer so I can spend more time enjoying the nice weather. And two, it keeps me busy during the winter, focused on something positive. The seasonal depression that hits me every year like clockwork hasn't seemed as bad since I began my writing journey. I still have less energy, my mood isn't as good, and I sleep a little more, but the cold winter months seem to go by quicker now than they used to.

    Even though it's been nearly six months since his thirteenth birthday, I still can't believe I'm the father of a teenager. Telling people I have a teenage son feels as foreign as telling them I'm forty. I have no idea how either of those things happened, yet here we are. The relationship I have with my son is great. For years, I only had him on weekends. Now we get together whenever we feel like it, which is usually at least two-to-three times a week. And we talk almost daily. Steph, his biological mother, hasn't seen him in over twelve years. I haven't seen her since that one Fourth of July over seven-years ago, but I'm still good friends with her brother, Chris. Sadly, even after all this time, Steph's still out there battling the same addiction-and-mental-health issues that have plagued her since adolescence. Though my optimism wanes with each passing year, I sincerely hope she somehow finds her way before it's too late. To be honest, I'm surprised she's made it this far. But I wish her nothing but the best.

    For the past few months, my son and I have been doing mixed martial arts (MMA) together. It's great for both of us, but especially for him. He's learning now what I didn't learn until I was in my thirties: confidence, discipline, self-esteem, humility, and the importance of having a positive attitude. Plus, it never hurts to know how to whoop a dude's ass if the need arises. What *does* hurt after every single training session is my forty-year-old body. But after living with Behcet's for all these years, achy joints and muscles are something I'm intimately familiar with. At least when they hurt after a brutal training session I know why. There's no mystery to that pain.

In addition do doing MMA/BJJ[1] together, my son's also been strength training with me since he turned thirteen. He bugged me for years to let him start lifting weights. I told him I'd start teaching him about strength training when he became a teenager. In the six months since we started, he's gotten a lot stronger and put on some muscle. You'd never know my son's only thirteen. I'm six-feet tall and he's only an inch or two shorter than me. It probably won't be long before I'm looking up at him.

I've never been prouder of anyone or anything than I am of my son. He continues to inspire me to be a better father and a better man. Everyday I thank the universe that he hasn't shown a single sign of having Behcet's disease. As far as I can tell, my son is a perfectly healthy and happy young man. And he's got a good head on his shoulders: certainly better than mine at his age. When I was thirteen I'd already been suspended from school twice, was smoking half-a-pack of cigarettes a day, drinking alcohol whenever I could get my hands on it, and getting into all kinds of other trouble. But worst of all was my attitude.

Fortunately, my son's nowhere near as negative as I was at his age. I inherited that negative attitude from my father, which he got from his mother. And I carried it with me for a long time myself. But since my son's birth, I've done everything in my power to break the cycle. By choosing

---

[1] Mixed martial arts/Brazilian jiu-jitsu

optimism over pessimism, hope over despair, acceptance over denial, love over hate, courage over fear, confidence over self-doubt – in other words, positivity over negativity – I've tried to become the best possible role model for my son that I'm capable of being. When it comes to attitude, *do as I say, not as I do* won't get you very far. You have to lead by example. And I've done the best I can to set a positive example for my son. I know I'm not perfect. There's always room for improvement. But all things considered, I think I've done a damn-good job. And I've got one awesome little man – who's not so little anymore – to prove it.

2020's been hard for a lot of people. Our country has never been more divided. But I've never felt better or more connected than I do now – and I have Behcet's disease to thank for it. I think a lot of people get caught up on the few differences we have from each other instead of focusing on the overwhelming majority of things we all have in common. They look for the negative in others because that's all they see in themselves. I used to be the same way. But since I've adopted a positive mindset and learned to see the good in myself, it's now easy to look past the differences and see the good in others. I've taken my overwhelmingly negative diagnosis and extracted every-single-fucking ounce of positivity from it that I possibly can – and that has made all the difference.

"Change is hard at first, messy in the middle, and gorgeous at the end." - Robin Sharma

32. Attitude

Attitude is everything. Luckily, it happens to be one of the few things in life we have control over. You don't get to decide where you're born, who you parents are, or whether you're born with a P or a V between your legs. You don't get to choose your height, how long you'll live, or whether or not to pay taxes (unless you're a politician or the CEO of a Fortune 500 company). What you *can* change is how you view these things. What you *do* have control over is your attitude.

I can't change the fact that I have Behcet's disease. If I could, I would've a loooooong time ago. But I *can* change the way I think about it – and I have. I now accept and even embrace the diagnosis I once denied. As much as Behcet's has taken from me, it's given me twice as much. But I'd never know it if I was still my old negative, pessimistic self. Developing a positive attitude has been like putting on a pair of x-ray glasses. It's allowed me to see the good inside every situation, every person, and even in the unlikeliest place of all: inside myself. Now don't get me wrong. Learning to be more positive doesn't mean all the bad suddenly goes away. It's still very much there. But when negativity is *all* you allow yourself to see, happiness will forever remain out of reach.

I've managed to find my own little slice of happiness despite all the pain and embarrassment I've suffered through over the years. I've learned to turn negatives into positives. My diagnosis is an obstacle –

not a roadblock. Sometimes I have to work around it. Sometimes it gets in my way. But I never let it stop me from living life the way I want to live it. Never ever.

Like anyone, I still have good days and bad days. Sometimes my joints hurt. Sometimes my brain is so foggy I can barely remember my own name. I have days when I don't want to get out of bed. I have days when I feel like anything that can go wrong will go wrong. There are even times when I just want to throw my hands up in the air and say "Fuck it. I'm done." But you know what? That's okay. As long as I dust myself off and try again the next day. Because each day is an opportunity for a new attitude.

We all struggle. We all have our own personal demons. We can only play with the hands we've been dealt. But it's not so much the cards we're dealt that matters: it's how we play them. Whether it's Behcet's disease, a different autoimmune condition, or some other physical illness; depression, anxiety, or some other mental illness; your parents, siblings, or other social circumstances – you can't change these things. What you *can* change is the way you handle them. You and you alone are in control of your attitude. No one can tell you how to feel about yourself, the world, and your place in it.

But that goes both ways.

You can't control the way other people feel. You don't get to decide what they think about you, themselves, or the world at large. Too many people get caught up in worrying about what other people think about them. I know because I used to be the same way. I would do *this* to look a certain way to *that* person. Or I wouldn't do *that* to avoid being judged by *this* person. But if you really want to know what people think about you, I'll tell you: they don't. Most people are too busy worrying about what others think about *them* to be thinking about *you*. So don't worry about what other people think about you. Most of the time, they're not. And even when they are, you can't control it. So why waste your precious energy worrying about what others think?

I like people. I care very deeply about my friends and family. I want them and everyone else to find happiness in this strange-yet-wonderful world. That being said, I don't give a fuck what any of them think about me. I really don't. I'm only concerned with what *I* think about me. I'm the one who, at the end of the day, has to live with myself. And after years of soul searching, self improvement, and attitude adjusting, I'm okay with that person. I like who I am today. I've learned to love my life – symptoms, struggles, and all. It might not be perfect. It might be filled with ups and downs. But this life I'm living right now, as far as I can tell it's the only one I get. So I'm doing everything in my power to make it as good as possible. If someone has a problem with it, that's on them. If someone has a problem with me, my illness, or the way I live my life, that's *their* problem – not mine.

Everything I've been through, all the pain and embarrassment, has made me who I am today. Living with Behcet's has made me a more-caring-and-compassionate person. It's made me realize that we all struggle, whether it's with an autoimmune disease, mental illness, or something else. But whatever you're struggling with, it doesn't define you. How you deal with it *does*.

I don't know what the future will bring, nor does anyone else. I have no idea if the worst symptoms of Behcet's are in my rearview or just around the corner. What I *do* know is that whatever happens, I'm going approach it with an open, optimistic, and positive attitude. I tried negativity and pessimism for nearly thirty years. You know where that got me? No-fucking-where. But since I've adopted a positive mindset, I've found meaning in my life. I've learned to see the good in this often-cruel-and-unforgiving world. Through all the suffering, through all the pain and embarrassment, I've managed to find happiness. If I can do it, so can you.

From The Author

    Thank you for reading! I honestly can't even begin to put into words how much it means to me that you took the time to read my fucked-up story. There's a lot I'm not proud of, a lot I'd do differently if life came with a do-over button. But that's how it all happened. That's my story and I'm sticking to it - because I couldn't get unstuck from it even if I wanted to.

    But I don't want to. Everything I've been through, all the pain and embarrassment, has made me who I am today. And I'm proud of who I've become. It hasn't always been easy, but it's been so freakin' worth it.

    If you or a loved one has recently been diagnosed with Behcet's disease or some other chronic illness, there are a few things I want you to know. First and foremost, you're not alone. Don't be afraid to go online and find others with your diagnosis. Reach out. Ask questions. You just might end up building some of the most-meaningful friendships of your life.

    The second thing I want you to know is that you and you alone get to decide how your illness affects you. No one gets to tell you how you're supposed to feel. Well, they can tell you all they want - but you don't have to listen. You get to choose your attitude and there's no right-or-wrong answer. Even when things aren't going your way, your whole body's sore, and everyone around you is in a lousy mood, you can still choose to remain optimistic. You can still look for the good in the bad, the light in the darkness, the positive in the negative. Sure, misery loves company. But so does the opposite. Positivity is contagious. You might be surprised by how your positive attitude affects others. In a world that is often overflowing with negativity, don't ever be afraid to spread some positivity around. It's needed now more than ever.

* * *

If you enjoyed this book, please leave a review on Amazon, Goodreads, or wherever you go to buy and/or discuss books. Every four-and-five-star review helps a lot. It doesn't have to be a long review and will only take a minute. Even just a few words are fine. But the more positive reviews the book gets, the easier it will be for others with Behcet's and other chronic illnesses to find it. To those of you who do leave a review, thank you very much!

Acknowledgments

There are a lot of people who played a role in this book that I need to thank. The writing, editing, proofreading: that was all me. While no one helped me to create the actual book itself, it never would've been written if it weren't for the people below. Hmmm, where to start. I know:the very beginning.

The first person I'd like to thank is Hulusi Behçet(1889-1948). He's the Turkish dermatologist Behcet's disease is named after. Dr. Behçet recognized it as a new disease and the medical community eventually agreed. In 1947, Behcet's disease (then called Morbus Behçet or Adamantiades-Behçet syndrome) became an officially recognized illness. While it's unfortunate that I'll forever associate your name with genital ulcers, thank you Dr. Behçet for being the first (in modern times) to recognize the disease.

In the years surrounding my diagnosis back in 1996, I didn't get along with my parents at all. But if it hadn't been for them, I might still be searching for a proper diagnosis. They made a lot of sacrifices for me, doing anything and everything in their power to help their sick child. My mother especially went above and beyond to relieve her firstborn son's suffering. I'm forever grateful for all the doctor's appointments she scheduled and brought me to, dealing with referrals and other insurance bullshit, all the copays and other costs, all the hours she spent in waiting rooms, the miles she put on her car driving me to and from my appointments, and everything else her and my father did for me. But mostly, I'm just grateful that they cared. I can't say that we always got along, but I *can* say that my parents always did what they thought was best for me, even when they really didn't have to. Now we get along great and have a wonderful relationship. Thank you both from the bottom of my heart for everything you've done for me, especially during those tumultuous teenage years.

  Dr. Scott Woods, as much as I remember you being an arrogant asshole at the time, I have nothing but the utmost respect for you now. You managed to accomplish what five other doctors couldn't: accurately diagnose me. Thank you for giving me the name of what had been wreaking havoc on my body since childhood. Though I haven't seen you since the mid-nineties, I've heard from a few patients of yours that you've calmed down quite a bit in recent years. Those who've been seeing you for a long time agree with me that you were very rude back then. I'm glad it wasn't just me. But they tell me you're much-more pleasant now, which makes me happy. Maybe for my next annual eye exam I'll come see you instead of my usual ophthalmologist. Again, thank you for diagnosing me, Dr. Woods. My symptoms fit perfectly. There's no doubt in my mind: you nailed it.

  I'd like to thank Dr. Masterson for prying himself away from his beloved garden that one Saturday morning back in June of 1997. You're the one who referred me to Dr. Woods at Mass Eye and Ear in Boston. He might've been the one who nailed the shot, but you definitely get the assist. Thanks for that. I might not have liked you when we first met, but I do now. I wish you nothing but the best - you and your garden.

  Dr. Burton Sack. I miss you and I know a lot of your patients and colleagues do, too. You were a good rheumatologist and a good man. I'm glad I got to thank you for everything before you passed away. Even though I already thanked you in life, I'll thank you one last time in death: Thank you, Dr. Sack, for doing whatever you could to ease the suffering of the scared, recently-diagnosed young man I once was. Your kindness and compassion will never be forgotten.

I'd also like to thank one of Dr. Sack's colleagues any my current rheumatologist, Dr. Raphael Kieval. My first impression of you was not a good one. But now I understand why you did what you did and I couldn't be more thankful. I appreciate everything you've done for me and hope you'll remain my rheumy for many years to come.

After years of unmitigated loneliness, feeling like I was the only person on the planet with Behcet's, social media has allowed me to connect with others who also have the disease. Facebook in particular has been amazing. I've made friends from all over the world who either have the diagnosis themselves or are the parent of someone with Behcet's. There are a lot of negative things that can be said about social media, but I'm incredibly grateful for it. Facebook, Twitter, Reddit, and other social media platforms have allowed me to, for the first time in my life, feel like I'm not all alone in the world.

I can't mention Facebook without also mentioning my Behcestie, Olivia, who I met in a Behcet's Facebook group. Thank you for being my Behcet's bestie, someone to share all my painful and embarrassing symptoms with. You helped me to live out a fantasy that'd been bouncing around in my head for over two decades. What a fun time we had! But my appreciation for you goes far beyond the time we spent together in Waterbury, CT. We've been friends for a while now and I'm glad we've remained close. It might've been Behcet's that brought us together initially, but our friendship has grown far beyond the boundaries of our mutual diagnosis. Thank you, Olivia, for connecting with me on a level I never thought I'd get to experience. You are and always will be my Behcestie.

    I should also mention Daisy since I dedicated an entire chapter to visiting her in Columbia, SC. You're one of the most all-around-awesome women I've ever met. You impressed me with your use of the word *tumultuous* (one of my favorite words) on our first date, again when you knew what Behcet's disease was, and about a thousand other times after that. What can I say, you're an impressive woman. Though our lives are going in different directions, I'm just thankful I got to spend the time with you that I did. I'll always reflect fondly on the time we spent together. I have nothing but wonderful memories of you, Daisy. And I'll never forget those big, gorgeous blue eyes of yours. Though we haven't talked in a while, I'm glad we're still friends on Facebook. I hope we remain friends for a long, long time. Thank you for being awesome, Daisy. I'll always care about you and wish you nothing but the best.

    Kady, my twin. I can't tell you how happy it made me to find you on Facebook. I'm glad you managed to turn your life around. Believe me: I know how hard it is. But we did it. We made it. Thank you for being there for me during one of the most-difficult times of my life. You were a friend when I needed one the most.

    Last but certainly not least, I'd like to thank my son. I've never been so fucking proud of anyone or anything in my entire life. You're my dude.

You've inspired me in more ways than I ever could've imagined. My little man isn't so little anymore. I can't believe you're a teenager - a teenager who's only an inch shorter than me! Every day you give me a reason to try to be a better father, a better man, and a better person in general.

Ellis Michaels Website

ellismichaels.com

Follow Ellis On Social Media

Facebook: @ellismichaelsauthor

Twitter: @ellismichaels9

Other Books By Ellis Michaels

Bad Unicorn

A medieval fantasy novel about a not-so-nice unicorn.

Ordinary Hero

A sci-fi gamelit/haremlit novel filled with adolescent action.

Inside Out (Bloodfeast book 1)
Back In The Game (Bloodfeast book 2)
The Final Quest (Bloodfeast book 3)

The Bloodfeast Trilogy is about 4 friends who get sucked into a video game – and their video-game characters get sucked into the real world.

www.ingramcontent.com/pod-product-compliance
Lightning Source LLC
LaVergne TN
LVHW051546070426
835507LV00021B/2426